TRUE BEAUTY

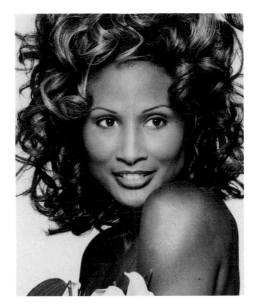

**Secrets of Radiant Beauty
for Women of Every Age and Color**

◆

Beverly Johnson

WARNER BOOKS

A Time Warner Company

Copyright © 1994 by Beverly Johnson
All rights reserved.

Warner Books, Inc., 1271 Avenue of the Americas, New York, NY 10020
W A Time Warner Company

Printed in the United States of America
First Printing: May 1994
10 9 8 7 6 5 4 3 2 1

Library of Congress Cataloging-in-Publication Data

Johnson, Beverly.
   True Beauty : secrets of radiant beauty for women of every age and
color / Beverly Johnson.
      p. cm.
   ISBN 0-446-51754-2
   1. Beauty, Personal. 2. Afro-American women—Health and hygiene.
I. Title.
RA778. J597 1994
646.7'042—dc20   93-47003
                                                              CIP

Book design by Platinum Design, Inc., NYC

◆

Foreword
by Whoopi Goldberg

Part I
Beauty: Your Inside/Outside Guide

◆

Part II
Fitness for Body and Soul

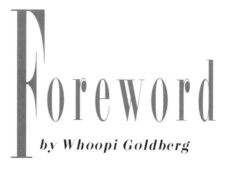

Foreword

by Whoopi Goldberg

Beauty is something we all want, and as young women it seemed so unattainable. It sent us into fits of depression and chocolate abuse. Not because we weren't beautiful, but because the acceptable definition of beauty was not applicable to us. When I was a little Whoop of a thing, the Breck girl was considered the standard by which beauty was judged. You had to have good hair—which meant straight, flowing and ponytail adaptable—light skin, and thin lips. If you were like me, you knew you stood a better chance of winning the Nobel Prize than of waking up beautiful. Then when I was a teenager, Twiggy and Jean Shrimpton set the standards, *and* there was Audrey Hepburn and that neck, those cheekbones, and that hair. Well, they were out of my sphere, too.

Then there was this huge explosion, or at least it seemed huge. To me, it was an amazing thing to see black women everywhere. Hattie Winston, with her little "afro," doing commercials. I guess someone figured out, "Hey, they must use soap and brush their teeth. I bet they even eat!" Then there was Diahann Carroll as Julia...beautiful, a single parent, with a job, on TV, doing what people do. And this was considered some sort of fluke or magical thing that no one could figure out. I mean, everyone knew that Lena Horne and Dorothy Dandridge were beautiful, but they were considered exceptions to the rule and therefore fell under the category of "exotic." But they led the way to Iman (whom they claimed they found running wild in an African jungle with some giraffe) and to beauty nonpareil Beverly Johnson. With Beverly, we were finally off and running, and the face that was considered beautiful began its slow change from, "Forget it!" to "Yeah, well, maybe...someday."

"Beauty" still has its ideals, but at least now the ideals are *fairer*. As they should be. We all know beauty shines from within but—come on, darlin'—when you're fourteen and full of pimples, or thirty-eight and full of crow's feet, it's a tough concept to embrace.

Times have changed from the days when we tried to find a shade of lipstick in the world of Petting Peach or a hair-care product when the only thing on the shelf was Lilt, and the idea that something was wrong with Dixie Peach Hair Grease and a hot comb. Or the idea that the GE Wrinkle Free Steam Iron was meant for hair, too. The days of being ashamed of the wideness of one's nose, the curliness of one's hair, or the thickness of one's lips—they're over. As a matter of fact, when you line up for a tanning salon, collagen lips, and Krinkle hair irons, they all lead to me. Except no one has bothered to put a label on that. That label is and always was "beautiful." Today, forget good hair and skin tone—beauty is where it should have always been: in the eye of the beholder. And when we look around, we find that we are surrounded by beauty. I'm looking in my mirror right now and I see a beautiful woman. I bet there's one in your mirror, too. Go ahead…I'll wait. Go ahead, girl…See? Now, knowing that, what can we do to enhance it? We start out by reading this book, baby, because whatever you are or are not—white, Asian, Islamic, Latin, black, and all the other shades in between—this book covers you. I call *that* beauty. And I call *her* BJ (Beverly Johnson), and she wrote this book for all of us.

Demystifying beauty makes us able to embrace it, and when your attitude is, "Yes, I am beautiful!" it becomes part of your thought process. It's true! You do feel better, you do glow. Now, it took me a very long time to get to that place because I thought everyone else was much more beautiful than I could ever be. It took me a while to change my concept of what beautiful is to include myself. So now here's a book that encourages you to get to know yourself and what may work for you. Because we are all so different, we have to take time to choose what's right for us as individuals. Have a seat…and read. This book is a gift. When you're done, encourage someone else to buy it. Don't give them your copy—you may start feeling adventurous and want to start practicing what it preaches.

Here's to BJ, from all the little girls who will never have to grow up in doubt. They will have the full knowledge that the judgment of what is beautiful is no longer in anyone else's hands but their own.

W (Hoopi Goldberg

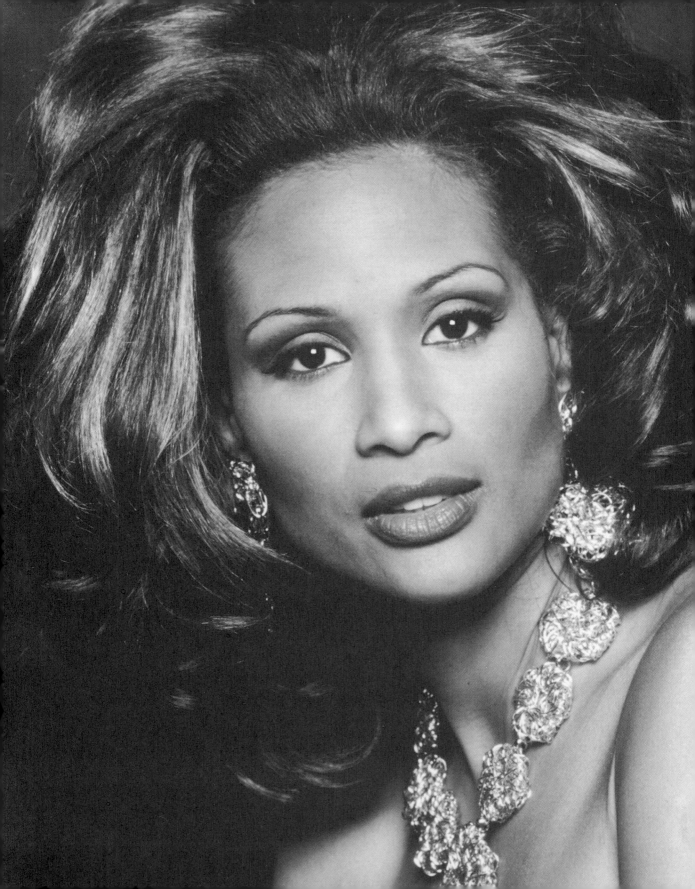

BEAUTY:

Your

Inside/

Outside

Guide

PART I

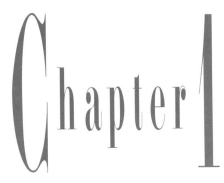

Finding Your Inner Beauty Center

What's So Special about You

For starters, there is a lot more to good looks today than simply putting on your makeup and fixing your hair. That "more" has to do with using your head. It has to do with knowing what works for your particular type of looks. Knowing how to evaluate the barrage of new ideas about makeup and skin care, hair, nutrition, and fitness, and the new products that go along with them. And knowing what your beauty priorities have to be, depending on your age, your level of fitness, where you live, and what you do.

Perhaps it's odd to be writing a guide to beauty these days when women are striking out in so many new directions and moving forward in so many new ways. But it's precisely because of these strides—there seems to be less time and more at stake now—that a sense of assurance about our looks is in order. Besides, this is more than just your conventional hair-and-makeup beauty guide. If there is one point that sets this book apart, it's that the achievement of beauty—*true beauty*—encompasses far more than the merely physical. It means not only the superficial attractiveness of your face and body, but the deeper, more fulfilling beauty of mind and spirit as well.

Mind. Spirit. Body. Face. True beauty comes from a complex interplay of all these things. Far more than a matter of the smoothness or color of your skin, the length of your legs, the

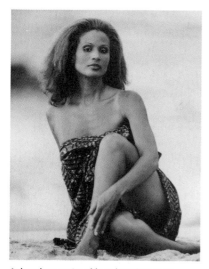

At long last, we're able to luxuriate in our own standard of beauty—celebrating the rich, multi-cultural heritage that's ours alone.

shape of your nose, or the texture of your hair, true beauty is the result of a harmony of many elements, inside and out.

Because this is a book designated for women of color, it's equally important to keep in mind that there is no single standard of beauty that defines the way women of color are "supposed" to look. Instead, in our features we proudly herald a rich, multicultural heritage—a beauty with its own vitality, its own allure, distinctly special, distinctly our own. In redefining beauty in new, modern terms—*our own terms*—we're celebrating the diversity of our coloring, the strength of our features, our own personal birthright of grace and style.

That's why, in the chapters ahead, as I talk to you about the beauty tools, the makeup techniques, the exciting skin-care breakthroughs of the last decade, the new, healthier thinking on diet, nutrition, and exercise—as they apply specifically to us, to women of color—you're going to find another thread interwoven throughout. That thread, addressing the crucial issues of well-being, self-motivation, self-knowledge, and self-esteem, is a key component to the achievement of true beauty goals. And I'm asking you up front: Please don't skip these sections. They're essential. They are—I'll say it again—part of what makes this book different from the beauty books of decades past and from the monthly how-to beauty magazines you may regularly read.

Perhaps you're already skeptical. But before you put this book down and say, "Well, I've heard about 'inner beauty' before, or 'I just don't buy that,'" please hear me out. Certainly I'm not denigrating the quest for physical beauty, which is something I believe *all* women, of every age, every color, from every walk of life, seek throughout their lives. There may be times when other matters take precedence, or periods in your life

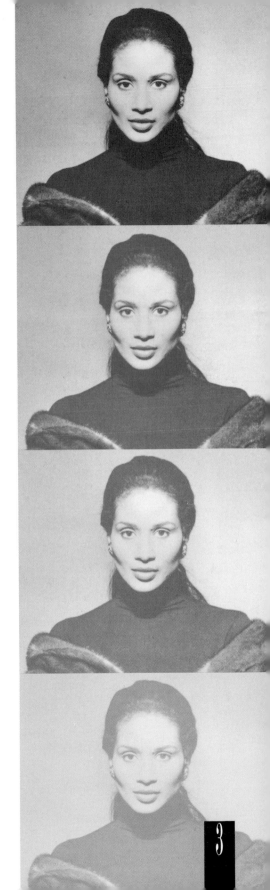

when this urge is suppressed, but believe me, no matter what people may say, it's definitely there.

But as women have moved forward—pursuing fuller lives, seeking better opportunities for themselves in the world, achieving better jobs, more fulfilling careers, and higher levels of education—many of us have also come to the realization that outer goals such as these are not enough if the nurturing of our inner selves is neglected. For example, as important as my work is to me, it's not the source of my self-worth. And it's self-worth that's the true source of beauty, both inward and out.

Today more women (and men too) are turning inward—we're taking the time to soothe our psyches as much as we do our skin, looking for ways to nourish the spirit as well as the body. It takes time to stop, to discover the things that make you feel good about yourself, *and then to go out and do them,* but it's worth it.

BEAUTY: THE POSITIVE PURSUIT

I firmly believe that the pursuit of beauty (both physical and spiritual) can be one of the most positive things in the world. Let me qualify that, though: as long as it's not to a degree where it precludes interest or participation in everything else. I'm certainly not advocating self-absorption, but psychologists have long

Realize this: caring about the way you look isn't narcissistic. It helps build confidence, self-respect, which in turn lead to achievement and the enjoyment of life.

3

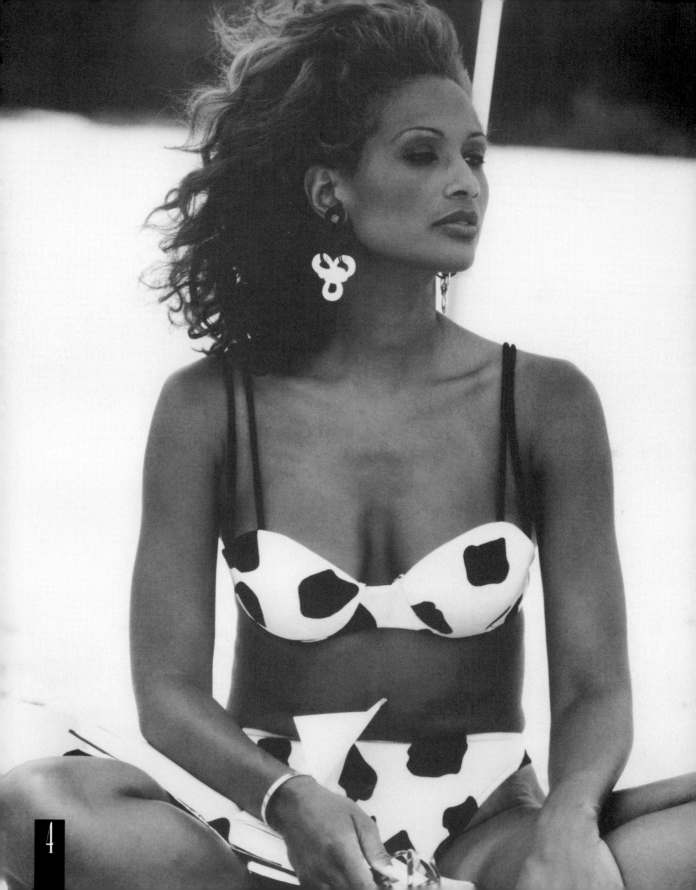

pointed out that the desire to reach your potential is an inherently healthy concept. All too often, unhappiness and self-consciousness about the way we look keep many of us on the sidelines of life, preventing us from trying to go forward and achieve all we can.

My beliefs on this subject come from having spent more than half my life in the public eye, as a professional in "the beauty business"—initially as a model, breaking the color barrier as the first African-American woman to appear on the cover of *Vogue* (and hundreds of magazine covers before and since), but also as an actress, an author, and a beauty expert, advising women on how to achieve their own best looks. (The topic I am asked about most frequently, by the way? Skin care. Whether you're twenty-something or sixty-something, that's every woman's number-one beauty concern. For answers, see Chapter 2.) But, like most of us, my life has other facets, too. I'm an active volunteer and a spokeswoman for causes I feel strongly about, like drug abuse and AIDS research. I'm the daughter of a loving, beautiful mother, and the mother of a loving, beautiful daughter.

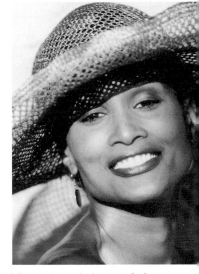

When you've made the most of what you've got it'll show—especially in your smile!

THE LEARNING PROCESS

Of course I didn't start out knowing about beauty. But because my face and my body became my livelihood, I've had to learn all that I can. Along the way, I've explored multitudes of beauty trends, sharing tips and learning secrets from other models, from the world's top professionals in fashion, makeup, and hair care, and from fitness and nutrition experts, too. In the course of my work, my hair has been straightened, braided, beaded, twisted, curled, and colored; my skin has been slathered with Senegalese mud masks, red clay, purée of avocado, and a stinging Australian tea-

Somewhere along the line, you have to make a decision about how much you want to work at your looks. When you do, that means developing a style that works with your features, your coloring, your schedule, lifestyle and environment.

leaf oil that turned out to be a mild skin peel. On one memorable occasion I was even covered—hair, face, body—with a slimy, dark-green mask of seaweed, purportedly to rejuvenate the skin cells, open the pores, and remove impurities. (The truth? I loved it, and when I was done, my skin felt—and looked—wonderful!)

But I've also had to learn (the hard way) to eat and exercise wisely. (Of course, I cheat now and then. My weaknesses: cookies and hot buttered popcorn!) Up until recently, for example, my battles with my weight have been constant. When I was a little girl, though, growing up in Buffalo, exercise was always part of my life. Extremely athletic since I was a child and thoughout junior high, high school, and even into college, I loved to participate in all kinds of sports—volleyball, basketball, and most especially swimming—all of which kept me fit. Once I came to New York City to pursue a career, I naturally became less active, and just as naturally began to gain weight—not great for anyone, but especially not for someone who was breaking into modeling! Since that time, I've attempted fasting regimens, fruit-juice diets, the usual salad-and-vegetables morning noon and night, and even a forty-day lemon, cayenne pepper, and maple syrup diet (I stirred those ingredients into fresh distilled water and drank it, three times a day!). I've gulped down thousands of vitamins, tried acupressure (though not acupuncture), rolfing, and Shiatsu and I've taken age-retarding high colonics and injections of lamb placenta.

Inevitably perhaps, I've inadvertently abused my body over the years by crash dieting and quick weight loss regimens. Weight *has* been my big obsession. When I

I share beauty regimens with my daughter Anansa, who's just eleven in the photo above. These days, though, we learn from each other.

was about twenty-seven, I went through a painful bout of anorexia, in which my weight plummeted to an emaciated 103 pounds (I'm 5'8"!). That was followed by bulimia, the painful binge and purge circuit. It was then that I truly felt myself slip out of control. My own body image and self-esteem sank to excruciating and debilitating lows.

BEAUTY—THE MODERN APPROACH

Today, though, I've come full circle, and I want to share with you the beauty conclusions I've come to. I feel the approach I've devised to beauty and health is a sensible one, taking into consideration my own personal experiences, and the many different roles that—as daughters, mothers, and grandmothers, as young women just starting out in the workplace, as homemakers and career women—we are called upon to play at different stages in our lives.

To begin with, I've always been a firm believer in a holistic approach to beauty and health. It's been gratifying to see—at last—the recognition and acceptance being accorded to homeopathic and herbal remedies, aromatherapy, massage, and other "alternative" techniques by mainstream beauty authorities. I know that ethnic women—African-American, Latin, Asian, Indian, Native American—have long felt an affinity with holistic beauty remedies (in fact, their practice is a time-honored tradition in our cultures). Shiatsu scalp massage, treatments based on fragrant aromatherapy oils, and the soothing point-of-pressure head and neck massages from which Japanese women have long benefited in their salons, for example, are now being introduced more widely in this country.

YOUR CHANGING BEAUTY PRIORITIES

Every age has its own beauty concerns and priorities, which is something I'll also be addressing throughout this book. As you enter your twenties, for example, you'll probably be building on and solidifying the foundation of beauty habits you established

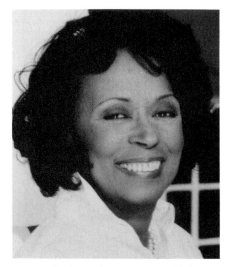

Every age has its own beauty. My mom, Gloria, reflects the kind of mature, elegant beauty that's confident and secure—the happy result of a lifetime of good habits...

during your teens. Sometimes the changes will be subtle, but important. As you enter the job world, for instance, you may want to wear more color, more makeup. Certainly you'll continue to experiment as you develop a more polished look. Your skin and your hair are now important investments in how you present yourself to the world. (**Note:** as you enter the working world, nothing does more for you—faster—than a good haircut.) Plus, once again, good habits now mean good looks, good health, later on.

What about women of color who are over fifty, or over sixty? I especially want to speak to you, my mother's generation, as well. Because it's from my mother, Gloria—a beauty in her own right, dark skinned, fine featured, so proper, such a lady—that I've learned so much about the meaning of true beauty, inside and out. Like so many women, I vividly remember watching my mother get dressed to go out—painstakingly putting on her makeup, adjusting the tilt of her hat, slipping on feminine, high-heeled shoes. She had, and still has, a way about her—a love of beauty and quality—that I know influenced me greatly. And her innate sense of elegance still manages to make the simplest things she wears look special...and beautiful.

It's to my mother and her generation that I want to stress how important it is to tap into—and hold onto—that singular and creative part of oneself, the part that makes each and every one of us unique and individual. I believe, and think many of you will agree with me, that there are no longer any age limits on looking well or being fit. While naturally there are differences (certain looks are terrific if you're under thirty, not so

...while Anansa's budding, young girl beauty is all about trying on images, re-creating fantasies...

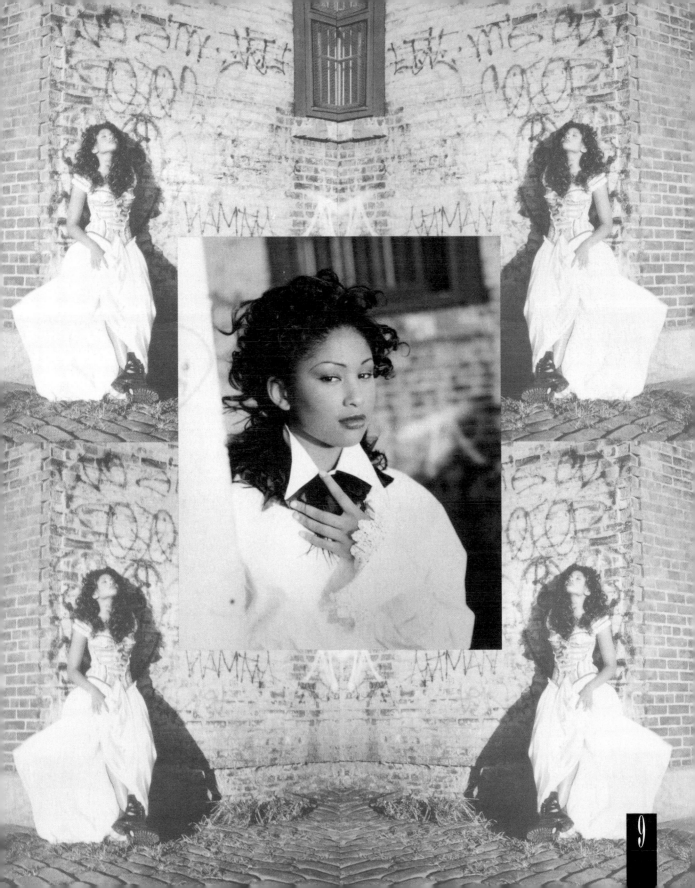

terrific if you're older), we've long since changed our stereotypical ideas of what "a grandmother" looks like. Today, grandmothers look sensational, paying attention to their bodies, their skin, their hair (shorter hair, by the way, though not necessarily short-short, is usually better at this point).

In and of itself, age is no longer—or at least it shouldn't be—the single determining factor of beauty. After all, how many of our most admired beauties these days are over forty, over fifty? And while each age used to mark a different moment of beauty for women, it's interesting to realize that today, even those traditional "turning points" are becoming blurred: "under thirty," "over thirty-five," "forty-plus" are meaningless labels when it comes to real life and real women. In short, while your age is the framework that helps you decide what's appropriate and what's not, you really have to look beyond age to find your own best look.

If you've got your priorities straight, you can easily get past the idea of taking it all too seriously and just sit back and enjoy it.

Today more women than ever before (whether by necessity or by desire) are juggling work and family, and working outside the home. According to the U.S. Bureau of Labor Statistics, there will be 6.9 million black women ages sixteen through forty-nine in the workplace by the year 2000—that's an increase of 23 percent from 1990. As we enter the work force in greater numbers, we will be seeking intelligent, practical, real-life advice

There are no longer any age limits on looking well or being fit. My mom, Gloria, a grandmother several times over, certainly belies stereotypes of what a grandmother is "supposed" to look like.

about our skin, our hair, our body types. At no other time, in fact, has there been as much emphasis or as high a premium on looking and feeling our best.

In fact, I find women of color everywhere demonstrating a new attitude and interest in beauty and health care. We're putting more thought, more time, and real discipline into looking our best. We're increasingly open to trying new, scientifically based regimens of skin care, and consulting dermatologists who specialize in ethnic skin. There's more awareness about the special needs of our hair; more general acceptance of new and effective treatments based on natural herbs and botanicals. If you've got your priorities straight, you can easily get past the idea of taking it all too seriously and just sit back and enjoy it.

While certainly there are (at last!) more cosmetic collections addressing the demands of the real range of colors of African-American skin, the fact is that there is still a lot of mere lip service paid to this "color revolution." Nevertheless, we're definitely moving in the right direction. There now are more makeup formulations than ever designed to suit our beautiful color-enriched skin, with all its light and dark highlights and undertones. For example, one major change over the last decade has been in concealers and foundations, involving the elimination or lessening of the amount of titanium dioxide used, or the substitution of a new translucent version (titanium dioxide is a white pigment that tends to turn chalky on deeper-toned

WHO THIS BOOK IS FOR

Of course, caring about good looks and wanting to reach one's potential is a matter of concern to all women. I believe it simply makes good, practical sense to want to appear at your best. But I've specifically directed this book to the distinct cultural preferences and beauty concerns of those of us whom society designates as "ethnic women"—women of color: Latin women with rich olive and warm brown complexions and lush, dark, wavy hair. Women of Asian ancestry, whose skin tones glow from pale ivory to subtle amber. African-American women in all our diversity, our skin ranging from pale golden almond to bronze to deep plum-black shades, our hair varying in texture from tight curls to soft waves. Although all Americans of African descent are described as African-American or black, the proportion of African ancestry varies from individual to individual, which accounts for the diverse and unique beauty of our looks.

But why a special book? Quite simply because no book has adequately addressed our specific beauty needs in a modern, sophisticated, and up-to-date way. For so many years we've been relegated to a once-in-a-while "makeover" in the women's magazines, and to a separate chapter or a page, indeed

11

sometimes only a paragraph, in conventional beauty guides.

Partly because we've been ignored (and partly because for years there was such a limited selection of beauty products geared toward women of color), many of us are just learning about the tools and techniques of makeup that enhance our skin tones, about the need for moisturizers and sun protection, about how to prevent hair damage and breakage from chemical treatments and processing, and most especially about the importance of proper nutrition and exercise, not only for beauty but for our health. In fact, there is a recognized health-care crisis in the African-American community, and diabetes, high blood pressure, heart disease, obesity—matters of increasing concern among our people—can be minimized and even prevented through education, exercise, and better diet.

On the plus side, the complexion of America is changing. The African-American population in the United States is growing rapidly and, with it, the demand for products, services, and information that address our particular needs. Teenagers—our beautiful young women, the fastest-growing age bracket—are most eager for modern beauty and health information. I see it when I visit school groups or talk to my

skins). There's also now a greater selection of deeper colors that flatter the richer tones of our skin. As a result ethnic women, especially mature women, who may have been disappointed in the quality of the makeup available to them in the past, are becoming more open to experimenting with cosmetics than ever before. I've even found that prejudices about makeup use have changed. One difference: The pales and brights, which ten years ago we were cautioned against trying, now can look as "right" as deeper shades.

But the fact that there are far more acceptable choices and more beauty options can be confusing in and of itself. There are any number of highly touted beauty systems, programs, and points of view; many of them work, some don't, and some may be self-defeating or even downright dangerous. There are more ways to exercise, more ways to diet (intelligently or not), any number of new makeup tricks, tips, and colors that are looking very, very good. The problem is finding the time to wade through it all and review it from your own personal point of view and situation, to come up with an approach that works uniquely for you.

As you go through the pages ahead, consider how these ideas can be applied to your life, your schedule, your personal needs. Some of you may be able to incorporate much of them as is. You may want to change other ideas slightly, in accordance with your personal needs (age, health, level of

To look your best, you have to know what your best is. This is me, with my dog, Flame, in my own jeans, my own jewelry—one of the looks in which I feel most comfortable.

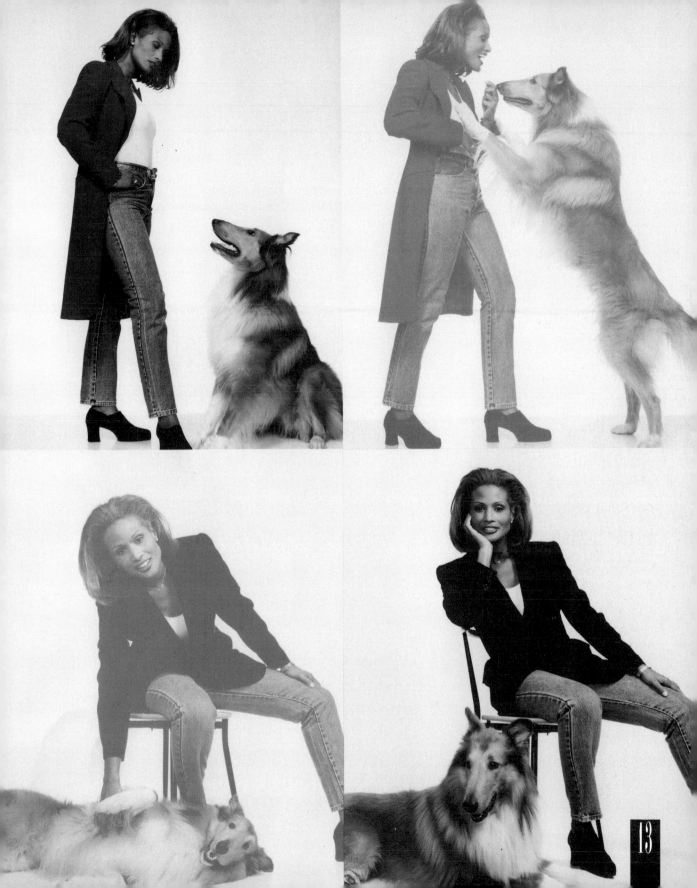

13

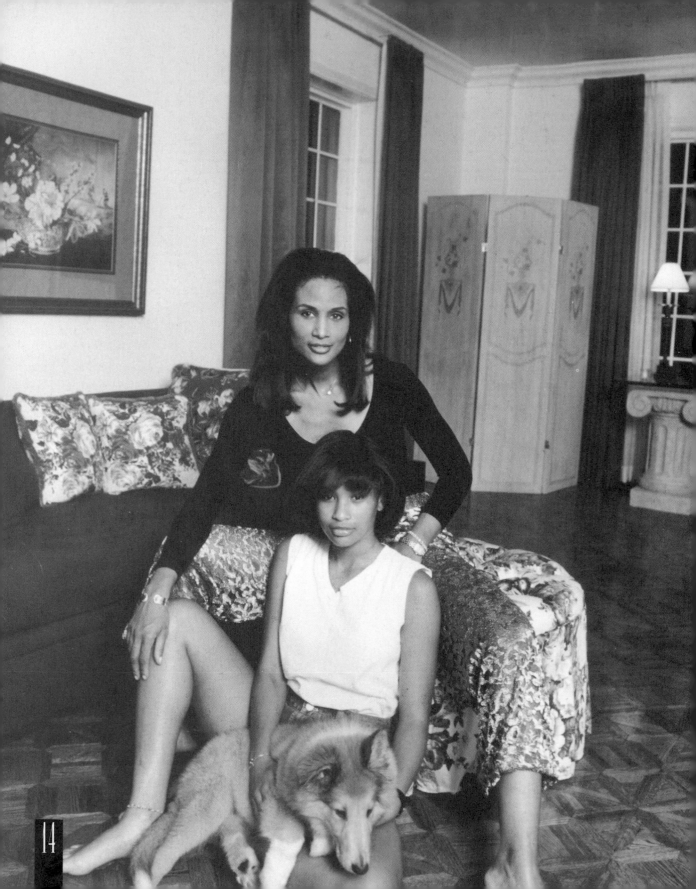

fitness, or the part of the country in which you live). The point is that while skin color may be our common bond, we all have different needs, tastes, and priorities that go way beyond race. Maybe you're a stay-at-home suburban mom with small children looking for time-saving and easy beauty pointers. Maybe you're an art director in a sophisticated big city; maybe you work in a high-powered law office; or you're a high school teacher in a small town, hoping to incorporate a new fitness regimen into your life. Perhaps you're a forty-something homemaker who already loves to work out, or a medical technician or a single mother going back to school, looking to take those first steps toward a healthier diet and lifestyle. Maybe you're already knowledgeable about nutrition and are just looking for some up-to-date pointers. Maybe you're a busy bank executive who wants a new look or a grandmother in her fifties who can't do a thing with her hair...

Throughout this book, my first goal has been to look for beauty systems that are easy to follow, and that are un-complicated and effective. But I also believe that beauty is a pleasure. If you've got your priorities straight, you can easily get past the idea of taking it all too seriously and just sit back and enjoy it.

♦

daughter, Anansa, and her friends, who, like all teenagers, love to experiment with new hairstyles and new makeup colors, and who are fascinated with all the latest fashions. And why not? Growing up, achieving the beauty and power of womanhood, is exciting. Plus, that's the age when good beauty habits and fitness consciousness begins, when the foundations of both health and beauty are laid.

Another "me" that I like: at home, relaxing with Anansa and Flame.

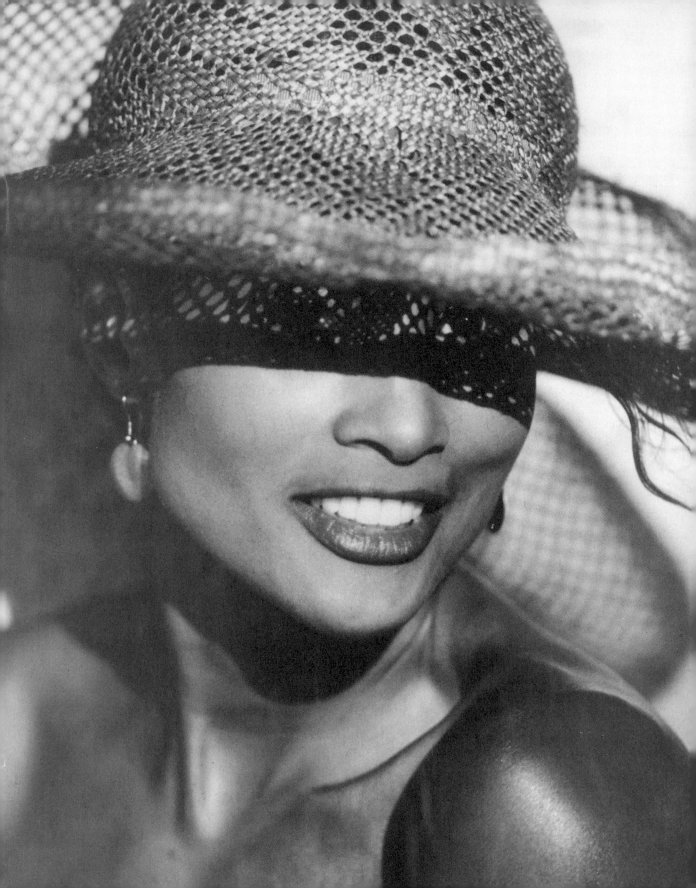

Chapter 2

True Beauty Skin Care

Solutions for Smoother, Clearer, Younger-looking Skin

Of course, true beauty is the product of what's happening *inside*—your energy, your sense of harmony, the strength and power of your inner spirit, all those elusive elements that add up to the beauty of the inner you. But it's important to realize that the inside and outside are inextricably linked and that the inner virtues you possess may not always be apparent to those around you. That's why the so-called "real you" consists not only of the inner you, but of your equally important flesh and blood manifestation as well. The beauty of the physical "outer you" flourishes only with care and attention.

Nowhere is that issue more apparent than in terms of skin care because, first and foremost, outer beauty starts with clear, smooth, unblemished, healthy-looking skin. In fact, good skin is not just a simple, routine beauty issue, but *the* single most important beauty issue for most women of all ages and all races. It's the beauty topic about which I consistently am asked, again and again. "What can I do about the dry little lines around my eyes and lips?" "How can I get my skin really clean?" "My skin is so broken out that I hate to look in the mirror. Beverly, what should I do?"

I'll never forget attending a graduation ceremony at Howard University in Washington,

D.C., along with a group of noted and accomplished African-American women (such as Maya Angelou) and being stunned when each and every one of them took me aside to ask me how I thought they might be able to improve their skin!

In a way, I think it's because our self-esteem—how we present ourselves to the world—is intimately related to the quality and condition of our skin. How many women, when their skin is broken out, have felt they'd rather stay home and hide than face the world? After all, if you've overindulged over a weekend on pizza or ice cream or other high-calorie, high-fat treats, you can (almost) get away with covering up those extra few pounds under an oversized sweater, T-shirt, or jacket. If you're having a "bad hair day," as we all do from time to time, you can wrap your head in a scarf, tug on a chic hat, or just sleek your hair back and hope for the best.

But if your skin has erupted—if you've woken up with pimples and ugly bumps—what can you do? It's really not hard to understand why some teenagers tell me that they'd prefer to skip school when their skin acts up. Women in their twenties and thirties often feel much the same way about showing up for work! The fact is that when your skin is terrible, you'll do *anything* to make it better…which is what we're going to be talking about in the pages ahead.

SECRETS OF GOOD SKIN— CONSISTENCY…AND FLEXIBILITY

There are two key things to remember when it comes to skin care. The first: that it's not something you can treat lightly, working on it today, forgetting about it tomorrow. Skin care has to be a consistent thing: You have to develop a regimen that works for your skin and then just do it—every day, morning and night. The second thing: Remember that it takes time to see results (nothing happens overnight) and that quality treatment requires constant, intelligent effort.

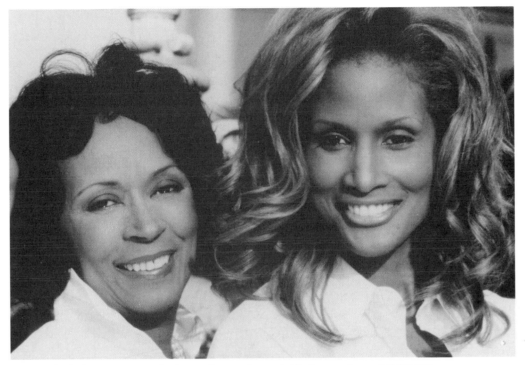

Good skin for the long term: no question it comes from good genes, but it also comes from smart skin care.

If you're a reader of beauty magazines, you might think that words like "care," "treatment," "system," and "regimen" are overused (and perhaps you're right). But the fact is that the ideas behind these words have never been more valid. I want to add another word to your skin-care vocabulary, however, and that word is "flexible." A flexible system of cleansing and care, one that is geared to your particular skin type and that changes as your skin changes, is truly what determines good looks. One is just not possible without the other.

Notice how strongly I'm emphasizing *flexible* here. Contrary to what a lot of beauty experts have espoused in the past, you can't just divide skin into types—like "dry," "oily,"

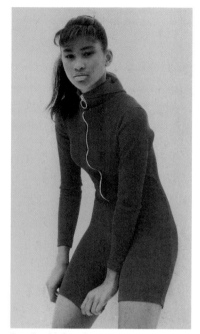

One nice side benefit to excercise is the glow it gives your skin!

or even that convenient catch-all, "combination"—and leave it at that. This applies to all skin, no matter what its color. The fact is that your skin changes, sometimes on a daily basis, depending on the climate, the season, the altitude, the foods you're eating, your health, even the amount of activity or stress in your life. For example, if you've recently been on an airline flight, your normally oily skin may be somewhat dry; if you're tense or anxious, or even if you just stayed up unusually late, your state of mind and your altered schedule will show on your skin.

Keep in mind that change also can mean positive changes: When you're pregnant, your hormones can cause a reaction (usually a good one) in your skin. And your skin will usually improve when you start to exercise on a regular basis (a nice side benefit!). I know that whenever I start a new exercise program that really starts my blood racing, I always notice a difference in my skin. In fact, if I know I'm going to be in front of the camera, the day before I'll even make it a point to jog three or four miles to make my skin glow and my eyes bright. Exercise revs up your circulation (the more you sweat, the better!), opens up your pores, even stimulates your scalp! And the results show up almost immediately in your skin.

FINDING YOUR BEST SKIN-CARE SYSTEM

Although I've been fortunate enough not to have major skin problems, the fact is that my skin does go through an unusual amount of wear and tear, with all the makeup I have to put on and take off. Because as a model I have to depend on my skin, I've made it a point to learn as much as I can from skin-care experts and people in the beauty business—from dermatologists, makeup artists, and other models with whom I've worked. Makeup artist Way Bandy, for example, taught me how important it is to remove one's eye makeup *gently*—not with a cotton ball, but with a cotton swab—because the skin around the eye is so delicate. More about this—the all-important best way to remove eye makeup—below. And it was when I was on a modeling job in Morocco that I learned about the emergency healing properties of toothpaste! One morning I got a terrible pimple on my cheek, which our makeup artist dabbed with a spot of toothpaste. I was skeptical, but two days later the blemish was gone. It's when you get stuck in out-of-the-way places and don't have conventional beauty aids on hand that these quick tricks of the trade come in handy.

Over the years I've experimented with all kinds of skin treatments. At one point, I even had a wonderful placenta-based moisturizer made for me in a New York City salon. It's interesting that through years of trial and error, my instincts usually bring me back to the simple, natural substances traditionally used as skin nourishers by women of color throughout the ages—cocoa butter, baby oils, petroleum jelly to smooth on body skin, hands, legs, all good, basic, overall skin treatments. As it happens, these substances actually do protect skin against the elements—chapping cold and wind, heat and damaging sunlight, all of which can age skin prematurely by robbing it of needed moisture.

How to:

First, remove your eye makeup with a cotton swab (sometimes tissue or even cotton balls can be too rough on the delicate skin around the eyes) and an oil-free makeup remover. (Be especially careful when it comes to taking off mascara—for special tips on that, see page 90.) Next, use a non-oily cold cream and tissue or cotton balls to remove the surface color of your foundation and any remaining eyeshadow or lip color. Follow up with a warm-water rinse (splash on with a coarse washcloth for a little gentle skin sloughing). After drying your face, dab on the moisturizer of your choice and, if you like, a little petroleum jelly around the eye area (I like to do this especially if I've been traveling a good deal and the skin around my eyes seems dry). • Another good way to remove eye makeup is with a natural oil, like almond or peanut oil on a cotton swab. Nice added benefit: The oil helps to condition your eye lashes!

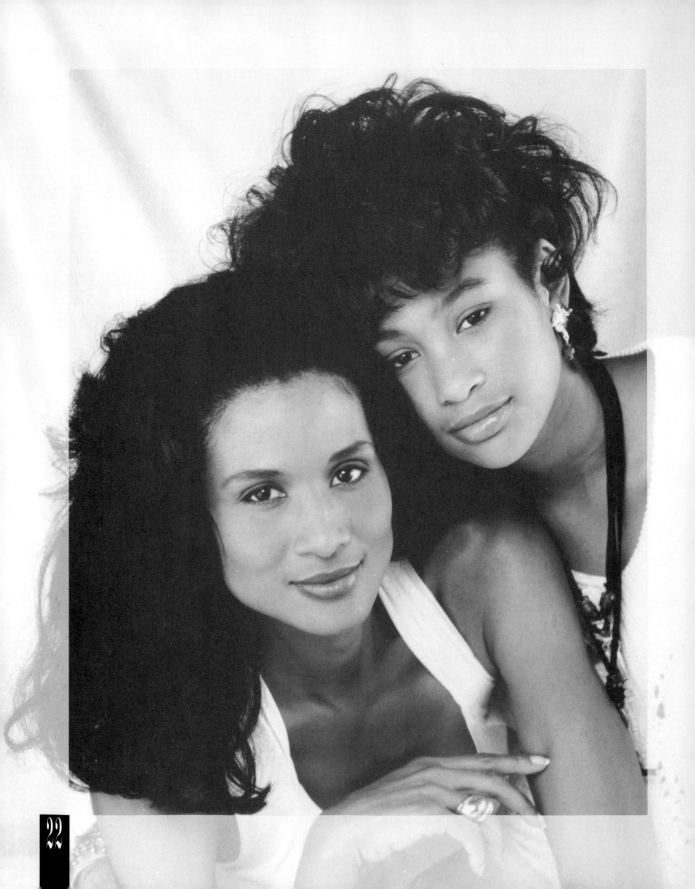

At health spas, where I go from time to time for essential rest, relaxation, and beauty boosting, I picked up the habit of slathering my hands in emollient creams, then covering them with little white cotton gloves to let the crucial moisturizing and softening elements really sink in. Taking a cue from many professional facialists, who always use steam to open the pores and infuse the skin with moisture, I've developed my own herb-laced face-steaming rituals, with fragrant herbs such as goldenseal and rose hips (add herbs to a pot of boiling water and steam your face to deep-cleanse, open pores, and revive circulation). In fact, steaming is one of my all-time favorite beauty treatments: Your skin simply can't get too much moisture! For a double beauty treatment after a good workout at your local health club, try massaging some of your favorite conditioner into your hair, then sit in the steam room for twenty minutes so it really soaks in. Your skin *and* hair will benefit.

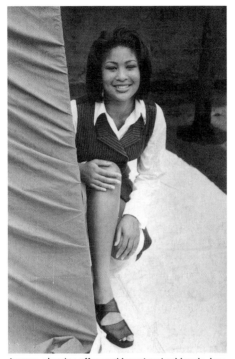

Anansa—showing off smoothly moisturized hands, legs.

I've also always had a special affinity for using natural foods and fresh herbs as beauty boosters—something I wrote about at great length in my first beauty book. I've always loved and recommended using such ingredients as acid fruits (strawberries, lemons, grapefruits and tomatoes) as a balm on oily skin. A slice of lemon, for example, is a wonderful, natural astringent for oily skin. Or place a tomato slice over a blemish for ten minutes to help remove impurities and spur healing. Oil-rich fruits, on the other hand, such as avocados, peaches, pears, or figs, are ideal moisturizers for medium and dry skin. Here are some of my still-favorite natural beauty secrets and home remedies:

Whatever your age, your skin can't get enough moisture. This shot was taken right *before* an *Essence* magazine shoot...and right after an herb-laced face steaming for both of us.

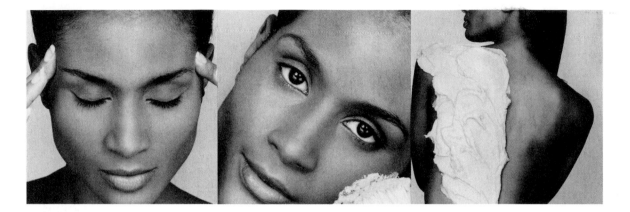

Thorough cleansing, that lets the blood flow, and brings nutrients and oxygen to the skin's surface, can help your skin look younger than its years.

- For a great under-eye cream, break open a capsule of vitamin E and dab it on. It'll help reduce wrinkling.
- Try taking 250 milligrams of niacin before a special evening out (I always do this before an important shoot), to make your eyes sparkle and your skin glow.
- One of my favorite masks for oily skin is to mix one egg white with 1/2 teaspoon lemon juice. Beat and apply to skin with your fingers or a wide brush.
- To soothe tired, puffy eyes, lots of models dip eye pads in cool rose-hip or chamomile tea. Place pads over eyes, relax for five minutes.
- To remove dark under-eye circles, try a slice of cold potato over each eye; lie back and relax.

YOUR SKIN—AS INDIVIDUAL AS YOU ARE

Because everyone's skin condition is different—and changeable—you will have to pick and choose to find the skin-care system that works best for you. And although we're long past the kind of stereotypical "beauty rules" and "one way to look" thinking of the past (in fact, I hope we'll be exploding some old-fashioned beauty rules in the chapters ahead), there still are definite *guidelines* to keep in mind. Certain approaches simply work better than others; they perform better for more people. For instance, dry skin will *always* benefit from moisturizers; everyone, no matter what their age (even teenagers!), should use an eye cream.

When you do look for beauty-care products, in particular the ones you use to cleanse, moisturize, or heal your skin, keep in mind that there's a lot out there—and more than ever directed specifically to women of color. It means we have to learn to approach these products with new sophistication, asking more questions and carefully evaluating claims. Keep in mind that while there may be some fast fixes and quick tips (and I'll tell you what I know about them), in the long run there are no shortcuts, no super-cures, easy answers, or miracle promises. *And when it comes to serious skin-care problems, your own doctor should definitely be consulted—and his or her advice heeded, to avoid permanent damage to your skin.*

Cleanse Carefully. When you wash, cleanse your skin with an upward, circular motion, taking care not to pull or tug at the finer, more delicate skin around the eye area and throat. Some beauty experts suggest using a coarse washcloth—the kind you can buy in a dime store—to provide a gentle exfoliating treatment that won't damage your skin. Instead of a washcloth, some dermatologists also suggest trying an extra-soft or gentle buffing sponge. (Exfoliation, a skin-care word you hear again and again, simply means the removal of the dead

BASIC SKIN CARE

Basic care means cleansing (at least twice a day, morning and night), moisturizing (just as often), and sometimes using a toner, especially if your skin is oily, but not necessarily if it's on the dry side. Plus, even though African-American skin is less prone to burning, sun damage, and skin cancer than Caucasian skin, we now know it's not immune, so it's a good idea to use a sunscreen when you'll be outdoors.

CLEANSING

Ordinarily, skin color—whether your skin is bright, medium-toned, or a very deep, color-enriched shade of brown, or whether you're Asian or Latin—has nothing to do with the skin-care regimen and type of cleanser you use. You may like a fine-grained soap, a cleansing cream or cold cream, or a cleansing lotion—it all depends on your personal preference and how oily/dry or sensitive your skin is at any particular time. I personally prefer a light, non-foaming cleanser in the winter, but a slightly heavier one in the summer when the weather's more humid and I want to get my skin really clean (remember, be flexible!). Sometimes I even use a little cleansing cream to remove my eye makeup, as well. Another pointer: When you can, purchase cleansers (as well as toners, makeup, and other beauty products) in small sizes so that the ingredients stay fresh and effective.

Keep in mind that certain skin products, particularly those that are scented or that contain potentially irritating ingredients such as lanolin or mineral oil, can cause discoloration and patchy light spots on those of us with deeper, ebony-toned skin. Since these spots can be permanent, some doctors (my own dermatologist among them) recommend washing with a clear, mild, unscented soap like Aveeno or Neutrogena (or, if your skin is especially sensitive, Dove and Cetaphil). For the same reasons, many abrasive scrubs and cleansing grains can be far too harsh for African-American skin. All but the very mildest should be avoided.

Note: If you're like most people, your skin is probably oilier in summer and drier in the winter. While some African-American and olive-complexioned Latin women may have oily skin, as a rule more color-enriched skin tones are no more oily than lighter ones (they may simply appear more oily-looking because of the way light is reflected on their surface). In fact, since dry, flaking skin cells are more apparent against our deep brown skin, African-American women do tend to be more aware of dryness, especially in cold weather, and inclined to do something about it.

cells that build up on everyone's skin. Although invisible, such cells can make your skin look dull, dry, and older than it should.) **Special note:** If you decide to try a buffing sponge, do so gradually. Start by using it every other day, then build up to everyday use. After about a month, if you've experienced no irritating effects, you can probably wash with it twice a day.

One thing that may surprise you is that I spend as much time taking my makeup off, as I do putting it on. I've learned the importance of this from all the most respected makeup experts and, much as I dislike doing it, it's something I've rigorously trained myself to do. My skin has benefited, and if you make the effort, yours probably will, too.

TONERS

After cleansing, some people like to use a toner (also called a freshener or astringent) to remove the last vestiges of soap and debris from the skin. I personally consider this an unnecessary step, but if you like the tingle and feel of a toner, be sure to use one that's gentle and unscented (it will be less potentially irritating that way). In general, an alcohol-free type is good for more mature, drier-skinned women; use an oil-controlling astringent if your skin is oily or acne-prone.

MOISTURIZERS

Maybe you think a moisturizer is something that only "older" women need. Or maybe you think that because your

One of the benefits of consistent skin care—that your skin looks good when you need it to.

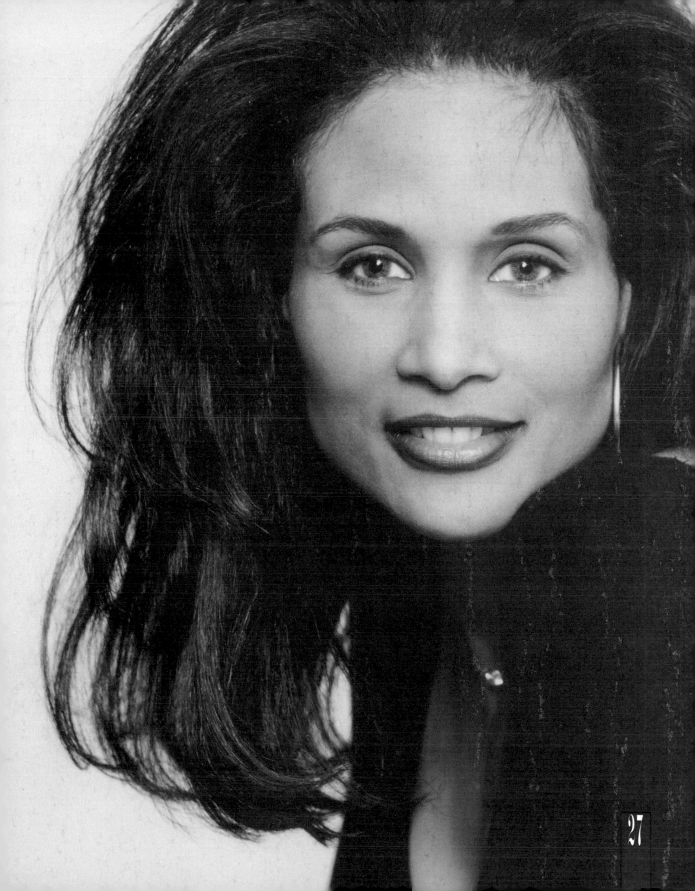

skin is oily you don't need one at all. If so, think again. First of all, moisturizers help the skin retain moisture—that's water—so the degree of oiliness is not a matter of concern. Second, dermatologists say that a good moisturizer is something from which skin of any type, any color, any age can benefit.

How should you choose a moisturizer? I suggest starting with the most basic kind—unscented, and free of lanolin and mineral oil. If your skin tends to break out, try any of the many oil-free brands; if it's dry, choose one with more intensive moisturizing benefits.

Once you've found a moisturizer you like (and there are so many good ones out there that I'm not going to recommend any specific one), use it religiously, and your skin will glow with the results. Gently smooth it on your forehead, cheeks, and throat in the morning and in the evening (dab a little extra around the eye area at night). If you're prone to a little puffiness under the eyes—common as you get older—be sure to dab on the outer corners only.

These are the basics of skin care, but there are lots of other beauty products that you may want to try. As I mentioned before, abrasives or grainy scrubs should be approached with caution by African-American women, because the patchy, light spots and discoloration that they can cause can be permanent. Washing with a coarse washcloth (or with a buffing sponge) really provides all the exfoliation our skin needs.

MASK MAGIC

Masks, on the other hand, can be a wonderful beauty treatment to indulge in now and then, as much for the emotional soothing they provide as for their beauty benefits. Remember, beauty comes as much from the heart, from the sense of well-being within, as it does from the physical. Applying a mask—taking the time to relax, to care for myself in positive beauty rituals—is an important part of my own true beauty formula.

I don't believe in using masks too often. Too many masks and facials, I find, simply promote wear and tear on the skin. At certain times, though, your skin may need that extra boost—a little deep cleansing—and that's when there's nothing as wonderful as a good, beautifying mask.

I truly find that many of the best masks are preparations from fresh fruits and vegetables that you can easily make yourself.

If you've been traveling by air a good deal, for instance, your skin may be dry and dehydrated, and a soothing, moisturizing mask may be in order. One of my favorites is also one of the easiest: Just take the mashed-up pulp of an oil-rich avocado and apply it all over your face and throat; wait a few minutes, then rinse. Nothing could be simpler, or more naturally effective!

Or if your skin seems extra oily in the T-zone (the forehead and down the middle of the nose), a drying, clay mask can do the trick. Or the egg white and lemon juice combo I mentioned on page 24. **Note:** When applying a mask, you can treat each area of the face separately: You don't have to use the same mask all over your face, especially if your T-zone is oily and the rest of your face is dry.

I'm not putting down the wonderful commercial mask preparations that you can purchase at the cosmetics counter or enjoy in a salon. But I find that many of the best masks are preparations from fresh fruits and vegetables that you can easily make yourself. For example, to give medium-brown skin a rich, coppery glow, try mashing a few carrots in the blender and massaging the purée into your skin. Another one of my all-time favorite masks is milk of magnesia! This is one I recommend applying at night, right before going to bed. Just smooth it on clean skin, let dry, then wear to bed; rinse off in the morning. The magnesia will tighten your pores, leaving your skin unusually smooth and soft.

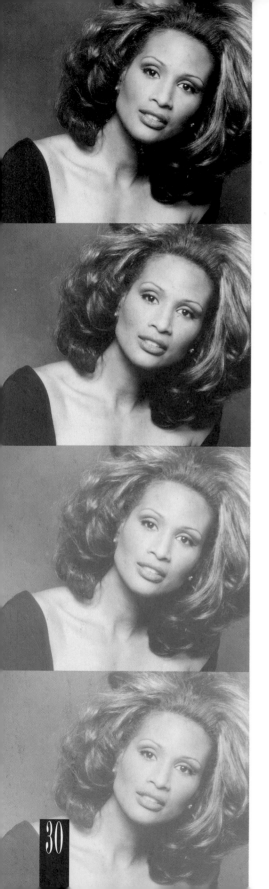

BEYOND BASIC CARE

These are the time-honored basics that you need to know. But there are other skin properties and problems particular to women of color that are important as well, and they can make a great deal of difference in the appearance of your skin. Plus there's what I call "crisis control"—tips on how to safely clear up problem skin, what you can do at home to give your skin that special boost, herbal remedies and model's secrets for at-home skin maintenance, and more.

BLACK SKIN/WHITE SKIN—WHAT'S THE DIFFERENCE?

To start, are there any key differences between black skin and white skin? The answer: as far as skin structure and quality is concerned, there aren't any. What *is* special about our skin is that it comes in an incredibly beautiful spectrum of colors—from pale, golden almond to bronzey suntanned shades to rich honeyed taupes, coffee browns, and sultry blacks, and everything in between. In fact, as is commonly pointed out, there are more than thirty-five variations of color for African-American skin (as opposed to about ten for Caucasian skin).

This wide range of differences in our skin color is caused by melanin—that's the dark pigment produced in our melanocyte cells. People of all skin shades have the

A gala look for a big evening—that's when we can play up the gorgeous, brown richness of our skin in a really dramatic way.

30

same number of melanocytes—about 60,000 per square inch of skin—but the cells are simply larger in African-Americans, and they produce more melanin.

Melanin, the pigment that gives our skin its rich and beautiful color, protects us. It allows our black and darker Latin skin to stay younger-looking longer by shielding it from the lines, wrinkles, and other ravages of chronic sun abuse that Caucasians endure. My dermatologist told me that he estimates that sun damage accounts for about 50 percent of the visible signs of aging in Caucasians, while African-American skin only shows about 10 percent of this damage. Skin cancer, thank goodness, is still rather rare among African-Americans, except for those of us with the very lightest skin. As for Asian skin, it ages much like white skin, but it generally tends to have fewer acne problems.

There are other differences that it's good to know about. For example, not many people realize that our skin tolerates cold weather less well than white skin, and consequently is much more susceptible to frostbite. Why? In cold weather, the skin's blood vessels narrow to cut off the supply of blood to retain body heat. What is known as "the hunting response" is what causes the blood vessels to widen again, preventing the skin from freezing. It's been found that black skin will reach a much lower blood temperature before this response occurs.

Ashiness

I've heard the term "ashiness" used again and again to describe everything from excessive skin dryness to the way certain makeup colors appear on color-enriched, ebony-toned skin. What ashiness means is that as dead skin cells dry and flake off (a perfectly natural condition, by the way, and not an exclusively black thing either), they show up pale and gray (or ashy) on deep-toned skin. • Sometimes, though, the word is used to refer to hyperpigmentation (or too much pigment on the arms and legs, which doctors find difficult to treat since body pigment problems are slower to respond to treatment than facial ones). Prescription-strength bleaching creams can occasionally help, but each case really needs to be evaluated individually by a qualified dermatologist.

Still another difference is that bruises and wounds heal faster with African-Americans, which helps prevent infection. Yet the same cells that heal quickly and that protect us against the harmful effects of sun and aging can sometimes act erratically to outside irritation or produce too much or too little pigmentation. That means our skin is prone to certain kinds of scarring and other conditions.

Keloids. Scars on black skin take longer to fade and have a tendency to "over-heal," resulting in thickened raised scars called keloids, which I know can be a cause of tremendous concern. When I was about ten years old, I fell and needed a number of stitches under my chin. As a result, I have a thin keloid scar that most people don't even know about. Keloids can develop from anything that breaks the skin: ear piercing, insect bites, paper cuts, acne, even minor medical procedures like the removal of a mole. If you're prone to them (and not every black woman is), they're most common on the body and along the jawline but rarely appear on the forehead, nose, or central part of the face.

> *Still another difference is*
> *that bruises and wounds heal faster on African-Americans,*
> *which helps prevent infection.*

If you know you're prone to keloid scarring, how can you can protect yourself? Before any minor surgery, let your doctor know you have a tendency to develop thickened scar tissue (I like to think that by the time I'm ready for cosmetic surgery, they'll have come up with a solution to this problem!). Even now, a dermatologist or surgeon can sometimes completely eliminate potential scarring by treating the area with an injection of diluted cortisone in the first month after surgery.

Hyperpigmentation. Hyperpigmentation refers to darkened spots or patches in our skin, which occur either naturally or as a result of an injury or irritation (such as a razor

These photos are some of my favorites. They were taken while the sun was going down, after a long day on location for a movie.

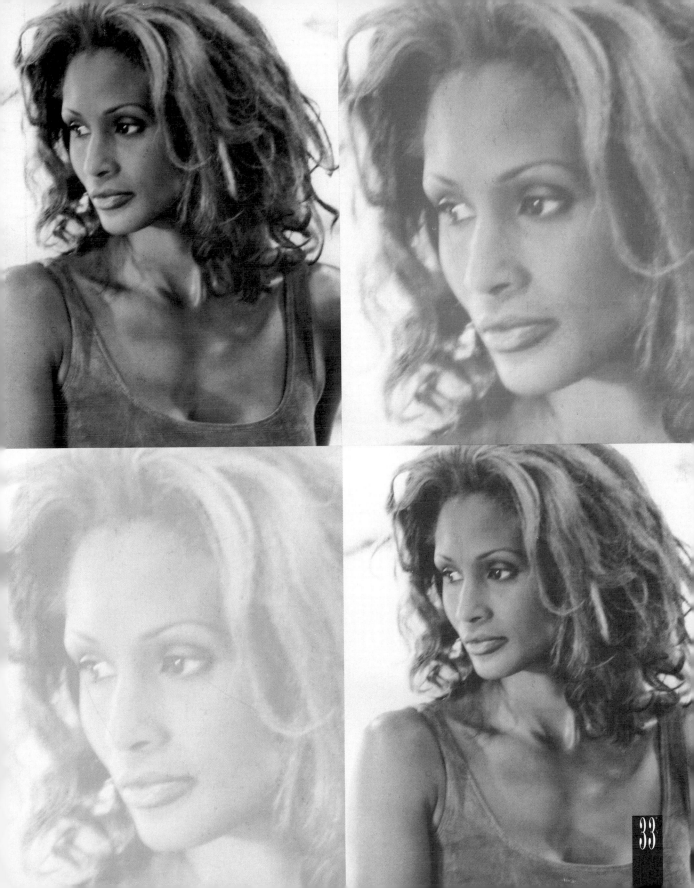

Bleaching creams

Most commercially available bleaching creams contain 2 to 4 percent hydroquinone. Those with higher content can irritate the skin, make the problem worse, not better, or even cause an allergic reaction. If you go to your doctor, he or she may be able to prescribe an individualized formula for you to avoid these problems.

♦

Keep in mind that bleaching creams must be put on exactly, covering only the spot that you want lightened. If you get the cream on any of the surrounding skin, it'll lighten that too. Try dabbing it on with a cotton swab for accuracy. And instead of a bleaching cream, for occasional unevenness of body skin color, try a little natural spot bleaching with slices of lemon or lime.

♦

nick, teenage acne, or childhood diseases such as measles or chicken pox). Since I'm athletic and into sports, I'm particularly aware of the scarring that can result from minor injuries and scrapes. After a year of using a bleaching cream, for example, I still have the slightly darkened scar from a leg scrape I got when I went hiking in Tucson.

Darkened areas may also occur naturally, particularly around the lip and chin, or on the elbows, the knees, and the back of the neck. They're most obvious on medium-toned skin like mine, less likely to form in very light skin, and they don't usually show at all on those of us with darker, more color-enriched skin.

Sometimes when these dark splotches are produced by an infection or an injury, they may fade on their own, usually within a year or so. At other times, they simply won't go away and need to be treated with over-the-counter bleaching creams. Before you use a bleaching cream, though, it's important to consult your doctor (see the box opposite).

I also recommend something called a skin toner, which has just a little hydroquinone in it (that's the principle ingredient of bleaching cream). I use this on occasion not to lighten but to even out any slight skin-tone imperfections caused by hyperpigmentation that I've noticed developing from time to time, particularly as I've gotten older. If you find you have a blemish or a dark patch, you might try one of these. Simply apply a little right on the spot.

In addition, many African-American women have naturally darkened areas at the elbows and knees, and sometimes right beneath the buttocks. If you don't pay attention to these areas—smoothing and moisturizing the skin—they can get dry and rough. I try to exfoliate dead, dry skin cells regularly with a gentle loofah (don't scrub, just lightly brush), and sometimes I use a very mild bleaching cream.

Loss of Pigmentation (Hypopigmentation).
Patchy light spots are another skin problem to which many African-American women are prone. For some of us, these are caused by irritating skin-care ingredients or by self-treatment of acne. Since these white spots can be permanent, it's best to leave minor blemishes alone and, once again, to avoid products that contain scents or heavy, potentially irritating ingredients like lanolin and mineral oil.

There is also a fairly common form of hypopigmentation that children and teenagers can get. If you're a teenager and such a white spot appears, it is probably nothing to be alarmed about and will most likely fade as you grow older. If you're truly concerned, see your doctor for a checkup.

Flesh Moles. About one-third of all African-Americans have "flesh moles" (the technical term is *dermatosis paulosa nigra*). These brown/black raised growths—about as large as a pencil point—are totally harmless. They're most common on the cheeks and around the noses of people over forty years old, and they often appear as you age. If they bother you, a dermatologist can improve them dramatically with an electric needle.

BEAUTIFUL BODY CARE

Because we all have so many things going on in our lives—work, school, family, recreation, and responsibilities—it can be easy to neglect the overall body care needed to keep your skin at its healthy and most beautiful best. I'm talking about your neck, feet, back, buttocks, arms, and hands, which are all part of total body beauty maintenance.

All-over skin buffing, as long as it's gentle, is one way to keep your body skin smooth, supple, and "polished." While I've already cautioned you about the use of overly abrasive scrubs, especially if your skin is on the deeper-toned side, you might want to try a *mild* honey and almond scrub, one of my personal favorites, or a Body-Mate by Buf Puf in the bath or shower to help eliminate dead dry skin and any rough bumps, and to gently (the key word is *gently*) smooth the skin on your back, your buttocks, and the backs of your thighs. Another natural body smoother is a little sea sand mixed with moisturizing cream. Please be sure that whatever skin slougher you use is mild. Any too-rough scrub, too-coarse brush, or even a loofah used too vigorously can seriously abrade African-American skin (that's why it's best to stay away from any scrub at all when it comes to your face).

What can you do if, as I do, you happen to like the extra-clean feeling you get from a scrub? It certainly doesn't hurt to check with your dermatologist about the merits of using one once every few months or so. Since everyone's skin is different, you just may be able to tolerate it. For example, I love—and have no ill effects from—the loofah salt scrubs I get now and then at my favorite health spas.

If you find you can tolerate a mild scrub, it's nice to smooth some creamy, lanolin-free body lotion on afterward to lubricate the skin and keep it soft. Slather it on your hands, arms, legs, back, and torso. Or try a skin-softening seaweed cream (these are available at many beauty salons). Plus, keep in mind that, like a facial mask, treatments like this have hidden mental and emotional benefits: the delight of pampering, the

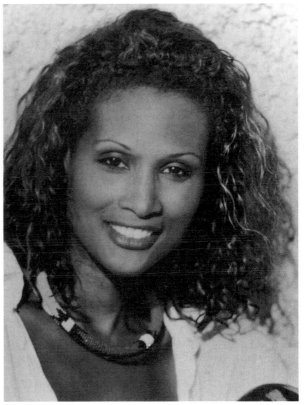

My hair—here's how it looks au naturel, just washed and dried (the African necklace is my own—a souvenir from one of my trips).

luxury of taking time to take special care of yourself. All of this feels very, very good.

Special Tip: If you get into the habit of giving yourself an at-home facial, apply the mask to your neck and throat as well as to your face (these other areas are among the first to show signs of aging). A weekly pedicure is also a good idea—not only for beauty but as a preventive for foot problems, to which African-American women tend to be prone. A good pedicure smoothes calluses and eliminates overgrown or ingrown toenails,

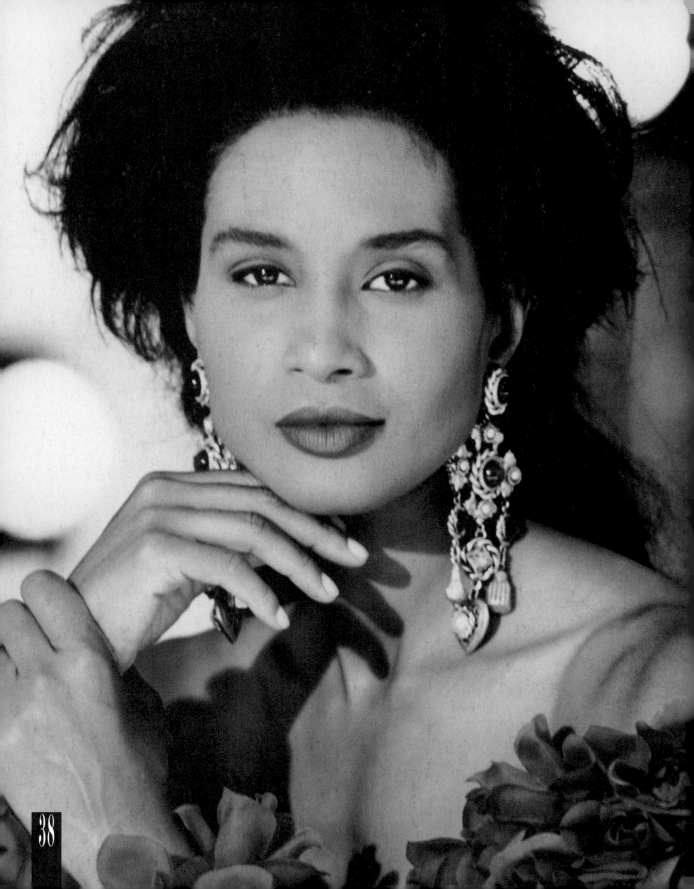

TIP

Real-life nail care

I love beautiful nails. In fact, one of the most important beauty advantages African-American women have is at our fingertips. Our hands don't show age as quickly as Caucasian and Asian women's hands often do (darker pigment protects against brown age spots and other aging signs). Plus some manicurists even tell me that African-American women tend to have stronger nails as well. The point is that if you don't have a lot of time or money to invest in them, all it takes is a few minutes a week.

♦

Basic how-to's:

Shape nails with a fine grade of emery board; metal files cause peeling and splitting. File in one direction only (sawing back and forth weakens the nail). Clip excess dry skin. Cream massage to nourish and moisturize, then clean around and under nails to remove excess cream and debris.

♦

Best nail shape and length: medium-length, slightly squared or classically oval nails—they're most flattering and most durable for most women. If your fingers are on the short side, a slightly longer nail will given your hands a more graceful appearance.

♦

Don't cut those cuticles! They provide a natural barrier against infection. Instead, massage with hand cream and push back gently with an orange stick wrapped in cotton.

♦

A coat of clear polish (practically maintenance free) will help strengthen nails and give them a well-groomed edge.

♦

When applying colored polish, use a good covering base and coat first for an even surface. African-American women with very dark skin and whose nail bases also are quite dark may find that transparent or light colors appear grayish on their nails. If that's the case, try two base coats or a soft, translucent beige for better coverage.

♦

Allow base coats to dry completely. Then sweep on two coats of nail enamel, again allowing plenty of drying time in between. Use three strokes for each nail; the first down the center, then one on either side. When both coats are completely dry, the last step is the top coat (apply to underside of nails, too, to help prevent chipping and to help your manicure last longer). Reapply it every other day.

Beautiful nails are just part of the story here. With extra-special earrings, sultry makeup—and a little bare skin— you've got a nighttime look that works for any woman, any age, when a little glamour is called for.

TIP

. . . Real-life nail color

Fashions in nail color change, like lip color or skirt length: Some seasons, bright colors are popular; at other times, berry shades or neutrals look right. African-American women whose skin has a yellow undertone should avoid nail shades with a bluish cast. Warm colors in the copper to bronze family, plus brilliant orange-reds, are generally more flattering. When pale natural shades are current, the look of a pale opal nail with a coat of beige applied to the tips can have unexpected charm against dark skin.

◆

If you don't care for polish, buffing will highlight the natural color of your nails. Buff gently no more than once a week or you'll weaken the nail structure.

◆

Are their cultural preferences as to nail length and color? It's something I've looked into. According to manicurists in salons that cater to an Asian clientele (like Salon Ishi in New York), Asian women seem to prefer subdued colors as most flattering to their skin tones. The manicurists at Ishi also observe that their customers keep their nails on the short side. Latin women, on the other hand, tend to prefer their nails long, Samy Suarez told me, owner of Samy Salon Systems in Miami. He says that many of his customers favor a unique method of polish application: The base of the nail and tip are accentuated with white polish, while the rest of the nail is colored a vivid shade of pink or red. "Spanish women are very meticulous about their nails. They'll even bring in their five-year-old daughters for manicures," he says.

◆

both of which can lead to foot problems. Pedicure how-to's: Soak feet for about a half hour in the tub, then go over the foot gently with a pumice to remove dead skin and calluses, paying special attention to heels and toes.

NEW TECHNIQUES

I've given you the basics, but I know many of you have other skin concerns. Because there have been so many new skin-care developments over the last few years, I spoke with a dermatologist for an update on their safety and effectiveness for ethnic women. Use the information below as a guideline, but keep in mind that our knowledge on these subjects is constantly changing.

Q. How should acne-prone skin be treated?

A. To treat acne and troubled skin, preparations (not lotions) that contain benzoyl peroxide are the most effective. Preparations in gel form, rather than liquids or lotions, are best, since gels are more consistent than lotions, which too often can become diluted, and thus less effective. One that my dermatologist recommends is Clear by Design by Herbert Labs, which is available without a prescription.

In addition, sometimes acne eruptions on the forehead and sides of the face are

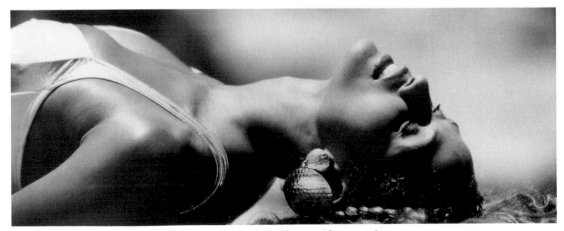

I love the feeling of the warm sun on my skin...but not too much...and *never* without protection.

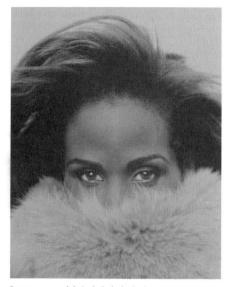

Everyone—models included—feels the same way: when your skin acts up, you want to go into hiding.

caused by heavy lanolin and mineral oils found in many of the hair preparations used by ethnic women. If this seems to be happening to you, stop using them immediately or switch to less-oily products that may help to clear up the problem.

What should you do if your breakouts persist? See a dermatologist immediately, before it gets out of hand. He or she should then evaluate your condition and provide you with an individualized cleansing routine, prescription-strength medication, exfoliants, topical antibiotics, and Retin-A or glycolic acid, as needed. While I'll give you a few of my own "crisis control" tips and in-a-pinch remedies, remember that nothing is a substitute for good professional advice.

SECRETS TO GOOD SKIN

• Fresh fruit and vegetable juices like wheatgrass, carrot juice, spinach, or celery, either alone or with meals, can make a big difference in the clarity of your skin. Plus they're better for you than eating a lot of raw vegetables since they're easier on your digestive system and enter the bloodstream much more quickly. Try a glass or two (or three) a day, and you'll see the results in your face.

• Step up your vitamin consumption (vitamin B, for instance, is a natural skin booster). So are herbs like ginseng. In fact, anything that's good for your circulation (exercise, for instance) is great for your skin and it will make it look alive, awake, and glowing.

• Water—make it work for you. Icy cold dips (in cold-water spa pools) can be terrific for your skin. At your local health club or at a spa, try going in the steam room, then the whirlpool, then letting an ice-cold shower hit you in the face. At home, splash your face with icy cold water twenty or thirty times to erase puffiness and swelling and to get up a glow.

• Smoking and drinking critically affect many areas of your life, but did you know that they affect your looks as well? They rob you of your God-given beauty (smoking, for example, takes away the much-needed oxygen essential for good skin). As for drugs, what can I say that hasn't been said already a thousand times? The self-destructive game of drugs has no place in the life of a person who honors her body and her soul. Drugs, smoking, drinking— all of these put up blocks and barriers to your spiritual growth. In order to stay connected spiritually, in order to make any attempt to reach your spiritual center, stay away. I practice what I preach—and I think it shows. I hope you do the same.

• Sleep—It's a natural skin beautifier. When I can't get in my full eight hours, I'll take catnaps to catch up. Looking rested shows in your skin—its tone, its clarity, its firmness.

• More ideas: A drying solution in blemish-stick form is a good thing to have on hand. Even better: If I find I'm really breaking out, a heavy, drying, pore-tightening facial mask made of clay or mud will usually help to arrest and heal skin eruptions.

Cellulite:

Although most doctors won't acknowledge it, we all know it's there. It's cellulite I'm talking about: the lumpy, bumpy, ugly "cottage cheese" that forms on the backs of your thighs. Although there's no cure for it, there are some "unofficial" things you can do to improve the problem. Since poor circulation and not enough exercise contribute to the formation of cellulite, start by taking a loofah and scrubbing down—really getting the blood moving in that area. When you come out of the shower, make it a habit to massage in a good moisturizer (slightly heavier than the one you use on the rest of your body). If you combine these two measures with exercise and the elimination of a lot of the fat in your diet, you'll see a definite difference in the texture of your skin.

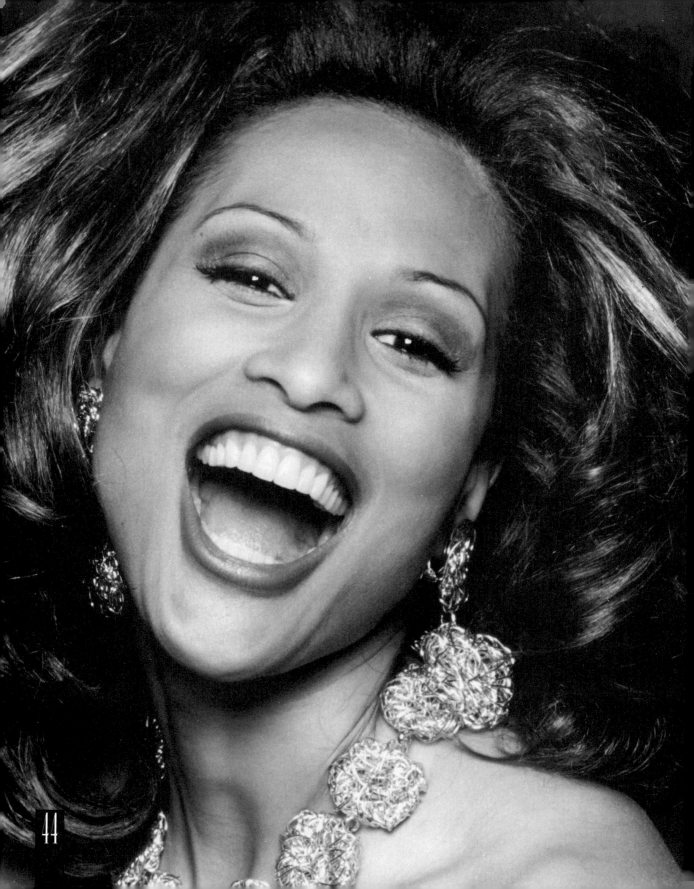

44

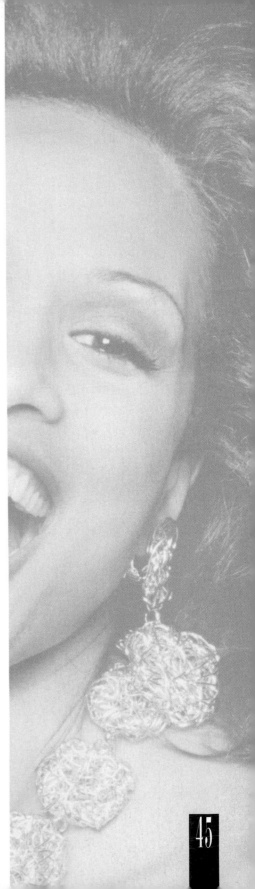

- What about blemish camouflage? Well, it's something we all resort to from time to time. One way is to dab on blemish cream, then put makeup on as usual, top with a little extra cover-up, pat down, and finish off with powder. Then, don't worry about it! Life goes on (even with a pimple!). That night, sleep with a little dab of clay mask on the blemished spot and rinse off in the morning.

- Although some experts may scoff, I also believe in the benefit of facial exercises, doing stretching exercises with my mouth, pulling my chin up, rolling my head, lifting my eyebrows. The face has muscles, and like any others, if you don't tighten and strengthen them they'll sag. In my first beauty book, I wrote about facial exercises, and I'll repeat two of my favorites here:

    To keep the jawline toned: Open your mouth slightly, and jiggle your jaw back and forth, left to right, four times.

    To firm the muscles of the neck: Drop your head back slowly until your eyes are opposite the ceiling. Open and close your mouth, pursing your lips into a kiss. Feel the muscles of your neck tighten and release. Repeat five times.

Q. Won't Retin-A or glycolic acid cause pigmentation changes?

A. Retin-A is an amazing synthetic vitamin A derivative that you can buy in cream or gel form, and that appears to

Your face has muscles in it, which is why it pays to do facial exercises. Like any other muscles, if you don't tighten and strengthen them, they'll sag.

reverse signs of aging, such as wrinkles, as well as fade age spots and freckles. While it may have a tendency to lighten (or darken) the skin, I am told that this is fairly rare and that your own dermatologist will be able to determine if you're prone to these conditions. If you have a tendency to hypo- or hyperpigmentation, of course, it's best to avoid them. Sometimes increased pigmentation will stop if use of the product is stopped; in other cases, bleaching creams with hydroquinone are prescribed to minimize discoloration. Hypopigmentation can also be treated with drugs such as psoralen and with ultraviolet light to darken too-light areas of skin.

These problems are said to not occur at all with glycolic acid.

Q. Is dermabrasion an option for black skin? Or does it discolor the complexion?

A. Doctors say that dermabrasion—smoothing acne scars by removing the top layer of the skin with rotating brushes—can be quite successful, depending on the individual skin type. It's sometimes even used to correct blotches of darkened pigment. The process is most effective in improving wide, shallow scars on very white or very

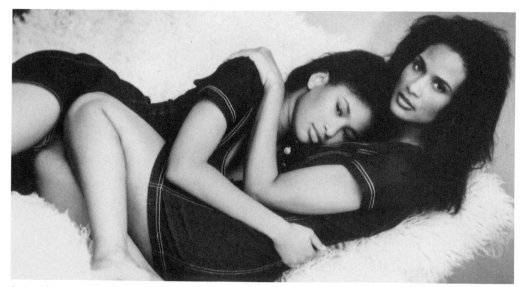

Just a quiet moment together...when I look at this photo, I feel that we're one.

dark skin. However, predicting the pigment problems that dermabrasion may cause on the medium skin tones of many Latin, Asian, and lighter-skinned African-Americans is much more difficult, and each case should be evaluated individually by a dermatologist.

Q. Will chemical peels cause a pigment change?

A. In the past, olive, brown, black, and especially Asian skin risked blotchiness (sometimes permanent) by chemical peels (even today, doctors will refuse to perform the procedure if they suspect that major pigmentation problems will result).

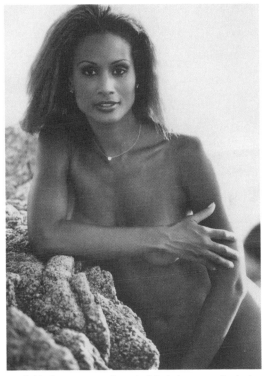

Good skin doesn't stop at the neck. It includes your entire body.

However, newer chemical peels that contain alpha-hyroxy acid are much gentler than the older peels, which had a higher concentration of an artificial peeling agent. They're certainly worth asking your doctor about. In general, chemical peels can work very well in repairing lines and wrinkles on most very dark or very white skins as long as caution is taken afterward (people with medium-toned skin are most at risk). After a chemical peel or dermabrasion, a 15-plus sunblock should be worn at all times for the first three months after the procedure, which is considered surgery. Direct contact with sunlight should also be avoided.

Q. Do bleaching creams really work?

A. Yes, to some extent, although one should be extremely cautious about using them (and always check with your doctor first). In general, look for creams with an active ingredient of 2 percent hydroquinone, and avoid brands that contain mineral oil. If over-the-counter products aren't effective, your dermatologist may try glycolic acid or prescribe Retin-A, in combination with a bleaching cream, to lighten up acne scars and other injuries without affecting the entire complexion. A dermatologist can also use a light chemical peel or cryotherapy, which freezes the skin with liquid oxygen, to correct problem areas.

If you do end up using an over-the-counter bleaching cream, experts say that if you don't protect the bleached area with sunscreen for the rest of your life, the dark pigment will resurface immediately. It should be applied carefully because if you spread the cream over large areas of skin, it could complicate the problem by lightening the light areas, as well as the dark areas.

Most sunscreens, by the way, claim to be waterproof, but remember that they're tested under ideal laboratory conditions.

Q. Do dark-skinned people need sunscreens?

A. Absolutely! This is probably the biggest misunderstanding about dark African-American skin. While you may not get burned, you're still exposed to cancer-causing rays.

Black skin does provide a fair degree of burn protection (equivalent to a sun protection factor of 10 or 12). But since most dermatologists feel that an SPF of at least 15 is necessary to guard against skin cancer, we do need sun protection when outdoors for more than forty-five minutes. Otherwise, you can discover the hard way that your skin can indeed redden, burn, and peel (it takes longer than fair skin, but it does burn). **Tip:** Apply SPF 15 sunscreen at least a half hour before going outdoors, since the chemical ingredients need time to penetrate. Smooth it on in a cool environment and reapply every sixty to ninety minutes. Most sunscreens, by the way, claim to be waterproof, but remember that they're tested under ideal laboratory conditions. If you apply the lotion when it's hot and humid and you're perspiring, it will run right off.

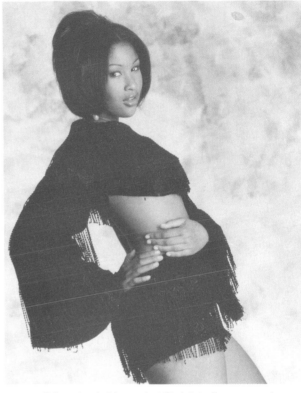

Anansa, all dressed up in fringe and a '60's hairdo. How you perceive yourself has a lot to do with how you come across.

Q. Does black skin react differently to plastic surgery?

A. Everyone is curious about this! Since African-American skin does have a tendency to lighten or (more frequently) darken after cosmetic surgery, question your surgeon carefully before making your final decision. Questions to ask: "Do you have other African-American patients? More than two? May I see before and after photos of them? Is my skin going to be lighter or darker? If so, do you have experience counteracting that? If not, will you be able to call in a dermatologist who might be able to correct

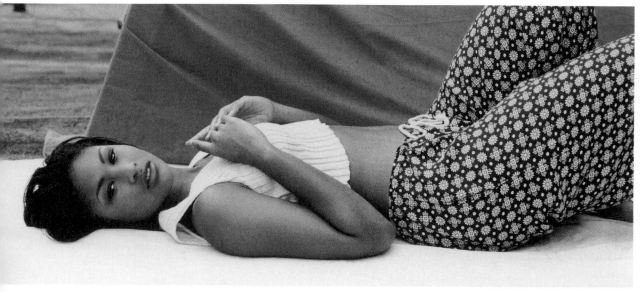

Anansa, in soft makeup, natural hair...and, a more pensive mood.

the color change after the operation?" Plus, make sure the surgeon is board-certified. A skilled professional's expertise will result in less bruising and keloid scarring. And read up on all your options. For example, many doctors are now prepping skin of *all* colors with Retin-A and/or bleaching creams before operating, which can prevent pigment changes and promote more uniform healing.

Q. What can be done about vitiligo?

A. Vitiligo, the loss of pigment resulting in white spots, seems to run in families. The cause is unknown. A dermatologist can treat vitiligo with a drug called psoralen that is exposed to a special type of ultraviolet light. But this treatment works only a certain percentage of the time. If it's unsuccessful, the spots can be disguised with a cosmetic, such as a Covermark product.

Q. Can the "mask of pregnancy" be cured? And what about stretch marks?

A. The darkening of the upper lip, cheeks, and temples, sometimes called chloasma, is a condition that's rather common in Asian and Latin women as well as in African-Americans (and often in Caucasian skin as well). It can result from taking birth control pills or from pregnancy, and is generally caused by a combination of sun damage, estrogen, and genetic tendencies. Going off the pill doesn't always make it go away, but a sunblock will keep it from worsening. How to treat it: Talk to your dermatologist, who may suggest an over-the-counter bleaching cream or a higher-strength, by-prescription-only version.

As for stretch marks, it's the rare doctor who will advise a pregnant woman to keep her breasts, belly, and legs absolutely saturated with vitamin E oil as a preventive against stretch marks, especially if your skin is on the lighter side. But an African model taught me this when I was pregnant with Anansa—I did it, it worked, and I strongly recommend you give it a try as well. Even if the tendency to develop stretch marks is purely hereditary, it certainly wouldn't hurt to try it.

BASICS OF DENTAL CARE

Where does dental care fit into a beauty book? Well, think about how important a dazzling smile is to the way that people think about your looks, and you'll realize that your teeth have a lot to do with it.

Dental problems, by the way, are generally not related to race or ethnic background (although I'm told that African-Americans sometimes have stronger bone structures than Caucasians and are less susceptible to dental disease). Proper home care plus three visits to a dentist each year are essential to keep anyone's teeth and gums healthy, and under no circumstance should professional care be neglected.

Some dentists believe that the addition of fluoride to our water supply several decades ago was a mixed blessing. While younger people do have remarkably fewer cavities than previous generations did (because fluoride makes the tooth enamel five times harder, bacteria can't penetrate the enamel and cause cavities), the fact is that cavities are still the main reason that most people visit their dentists. And because we have fewer cavities, we tend to visit our dentists less frequently.

The problem is that fluoride doesn't strengthen the gums. And, cavities notwithstanding, if you don't have regular professional cleanings, bacteria can reach between the teeth and gums, causing tooth decay in young people or periodontal disease (usually if you're over forty).

As we get older—into our forties and fifties—the bacteria in our mouths becomes more able to survive without oxygen and remains between the teeth and gums, breaking down the periodontal ligament around the tooth and attacking the bone. It's at this point that there's a good chance of losing a tooth.

Local teaching institutions and hospitals provide excellent care and cost less than private dentists. Some places won't even charge you for your third visit of the year, if you're a regular patient who's conscientious about home care. It's only when people miss appointments and don't take care of themselves that dental professionals won't reach out to help them.

> *A trip to the dentist to remove plaque—the sticky film produced by bacteria— doesn't have to be expensive.*

Ask your dentist or dental hygienist to show you how to brush and floss properly to destroy plaque. **Note:** Electric toothbrushes are exceptionally good at reaching plaque in the areas that flossing sometimes misses—behind the teeth and all the way back into the mouth. My dentist gave me techniques for brushing twice a day, and flossing once (see box).

♦

HOW TO BRUSH

Most people concentrate on brushing the outside surface and tops of the teeth, but the tongue washes away most of the plaque from these areas. You need to get the bristles underneath the gum line, at the rim around the teeth, and between the teeth where the bacteria hides.

Use a toothbrush with soft or extra-soft bristles. Hard bristles abrade the teeth and erode the tooth structure and enamel. For the same reason, avoid abrasive toothpastes that claim to make teeth brighter and whiter. Whitening can only be accomplished by chemical means. Baking soda toothpastes are effective at killing bacteria. Slant the bristles of the toothbrush at a 45 degree angle toward your gum line and brush across—not up and down.

HOW TO FLOSS

Gently pull the floss under the gum line. If you just pull downward, you'll go into the gums and tear them. Go down between each two teeth; floss one way around the neck of the tooth toward the front, then lift the floss up a little bit and go around the neck behind it. Use up-and-down motion, not a sideways one.

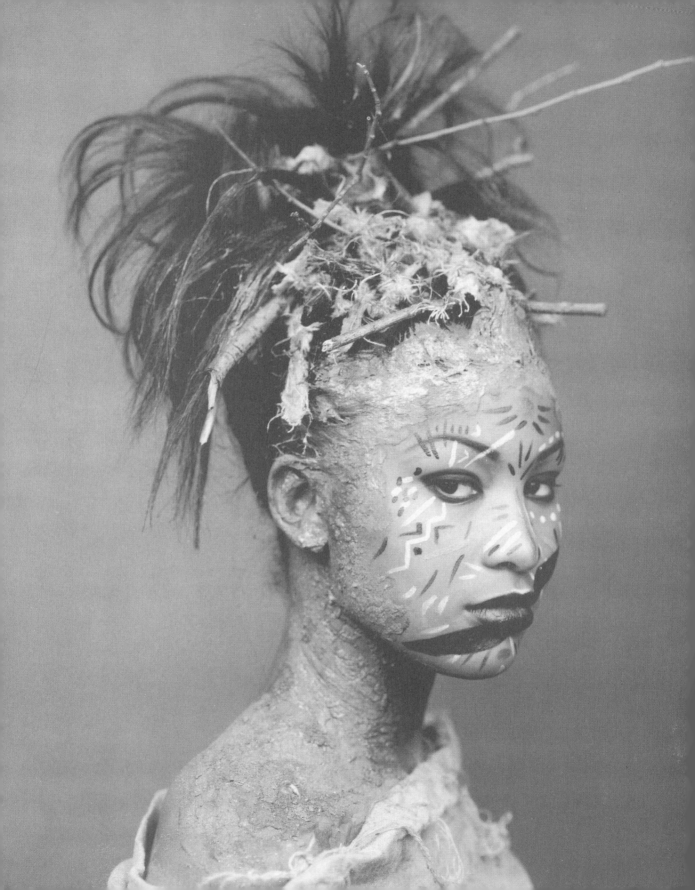

Chapter 3

True Beauty Makeup

Tricks of the Trade: Makeup That Adds Impact

In this chapter I'm going to talk about makeup—not in terms of step-by-step instruction that you should blindly memorize and follow, but rather in terms of timeless makeup principles that will almost always apply for women of color, season after season, year after year. Once you understand the ideas behind these principles—why certain makeup colors will always be flattering to us, what to look for in a foundation or a lip color, the most effective blending and contouring techniques—you can then apply them to whatever is "in fashion" at that particular moment.

Someone once told me that you have only one chance to make a first impression—that's how people will perceive and remember you, and they never really "see" you again. It's a simple thing, but it's something I've never forgotten to this day. What it reinforces in my mind (and, I hope, in yours) is just how important it is that that first impression be a positive one—if possible, a dramatic and individual statement that says exactly who you are. And the fact is that a lot of that statement can depend on your facility with makeup, not only the colors you choose, but also how much or how little you feel comfortable wearing, and how effectively you apply it.

Enhance cheekbones.　　　　**Full, strong Lips.**　　　　**Defined brows and skin that glows.**

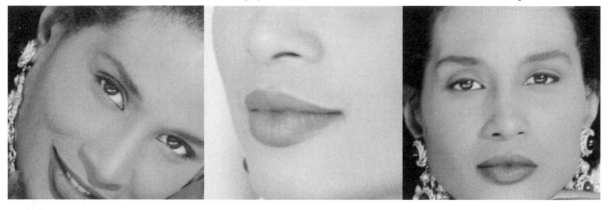

When I say "a dramatic statement," I don't mean harsh or overstated makeup. Far from it. In fact, the makeup I prefer personally on a daily basis is more understated than anything else. The best—and the most modern—approach is makeup that subtly enhances but doesn't change your appearance, playing up your assets and minimizing your "flaws." Anything more obvious can be instantly aging and old-fashioned.

This is what I find works most of the time:

• Strong but sheer colors

• A defined and shapely brow

• Skin that glows with a sunny, sheer finish

Of course, there may be variations from time to time. Some years, for example, you'll find that a matte finish looks newest, or a richer lip color, or a thinner, arched eyebrow; other years, you'll want a shinier, dewier look, neutral lips, fuller brows. In general, though, these are the basic makeup guidelines you should keep in mind.

Depending on your personality and the colors you use, your basic makeup may range from a "natural" look (not the natural, no-makeup face of the 70's, but one that's subtle, blended, and refined) to a slightly more theatrical effect. Either way, what counts is an attention to detail, to all the little things that add up to a polished, well-groomed appearance.

What's also important to know about makeup is that whether the result you're going for is soft or sophisticated, your basic techniques will remain the same: A concealer or color corrector of some kind (unless your skin is very, very good) will nearly always be your "first step." Your blusher will usually be applied in a certain way. At night while you may want to intensify the makeup you're wearing, choosing deeper or heightened colors—a charcoal-black shadow instead of medium brown, a richer plum-violet instead of lavender—or, adding a touch of shimmer or sparkle, the basic techniques won't change. As much as makeup can do for your looks, I have to admit it's actually your clothes and the accessories you choose that create the desired evening effect.

That's not to say I haven't seen women who've never worn makeup before whose looks were totally transformed by just a touch of color on their lips or cheeks (and how wonderful it was to see their confidence level soar as a result). Even among my colleagues—professional models whose un-made-up looks can range from simply pretty to rather plain— become absolutely dazzling as skillfully applied makeup highlights their features and brings them into focus.

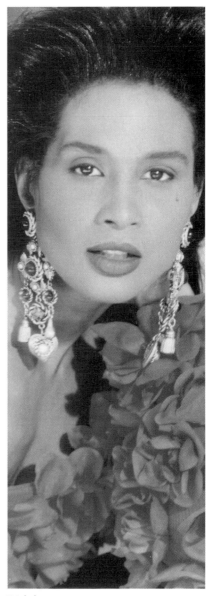

Total glamour makeup, hair, jewelry; everything works together.

HOW TO BEGIN

Starting out and no matter what your age, if you've never worn much makeup before, it's important to introduce yourself to its use gradually, choosing just a few easy-to-handle colors (mostly neutrals) rather than attempting fancy tricks or special effects. These are the colors that you'll end up wearing most often and that will serve you in good stead for years to come. Your goal, after all, is to reach a comfort level with makeup, and most people feel comfortable when they have the knowledge to back up what they're doing. Once you have that basic knowledge, you can certainly move on to more creative, more innovative makeup techniques.

Cleaning Brushes and Puffs: Because makeup brushes and powder puffs pick up oil and bacteria from the skin, they should be cleaned properly—ideally once a week, but at least every other week. When you apply your makeup with a soiled brush or puff, not only will the makeup not blend as well, but the colors may become muddied and dull. Cleaning brushes also extends their working life, which is important once you've invested in a good set. *How to's:* Soak brushes in warm, soapy water (a mild baby shampoo or liquid dishwashing detergent is a good choice) for ten or fifteen minutes. Then rinse, towel blot, and let dry naturally (for a quick dry, try a hair dryer on its lowest setting).

When you're in your teens, you probably will look best with a fairly minimal makeup that lets the freshness and prettiness of your skin come through. That's not to say you shouldn't have fun with your makeup and be outrageous every once in a while. Of couse, you should! But we're talking basic everyday makeup here. On the other hand, if you're in your thirties, forties, or fifties, or if you're a professional out in the working world, you'll probably want your makeup to be more polished and refined. You may want to accent your cheekbones more dramatically, for instance, or apply additional highlighter for terrific added impact, especially at night.

Whatever your situation, when you look at photographs of models in magazines, keep in mind that a professional makeup artist applied the makeup that you see. It took a lot of time and a lot of skill; it was created not for real life, but was specifically exaggerated for the camera's eye. In reality, most women would probably want to "translate" that makeup by toning down its colorings or changing its point of emphasis somewhat. Learn how to selectively interpret the looks you see rather than trying to slavishly copy them. Use them as starting points, as sources for new ideas, as clever tricks not to copy but to help you achieve a look that's uniquely your own.

Finally, no matter how proficient you become with makeup, remember that it's not and was never meant to be "the main event." Rather, it's the finishing touch. What you do first in the way of skin care and treatment is far more important.

YOUR SEVEN ALL-PURPOSE MAKEUP GUIDELINES

As you look at yourself in the mirror, there are seven basic guidelines to keep in mind.

1. You can wear any makeup color you want, as long as it has a sheer appearance. Even a color that's too dark or too harsh for your skin tone becomes instantly more wearable when you "sheer" it down with a little moisturizer or water.

2. Women of color whose skin glows with deep, rich, ebony tones do not need more makeup than their lighter-skinned counterparts; they should just use deeper tones.

3. The trick to good daytime makeup is for the color to look as if it were "born" there…naturally. Always apply makeup a little at a time, then blend. Remember, you can always add; it's much harder to eliminate color. (This is something most of us have experienced: When you make a mistake and try to remove excess, the makeup that remains tends to become smudgy and won't blend as well. Instead of saving time, you end up starting from scratch, anyway.)

4. We are people of color, so don't be afraid of using it. Because of the richness of our skin tones, we can actually use more color on our faces—color that's stronger, richer, even

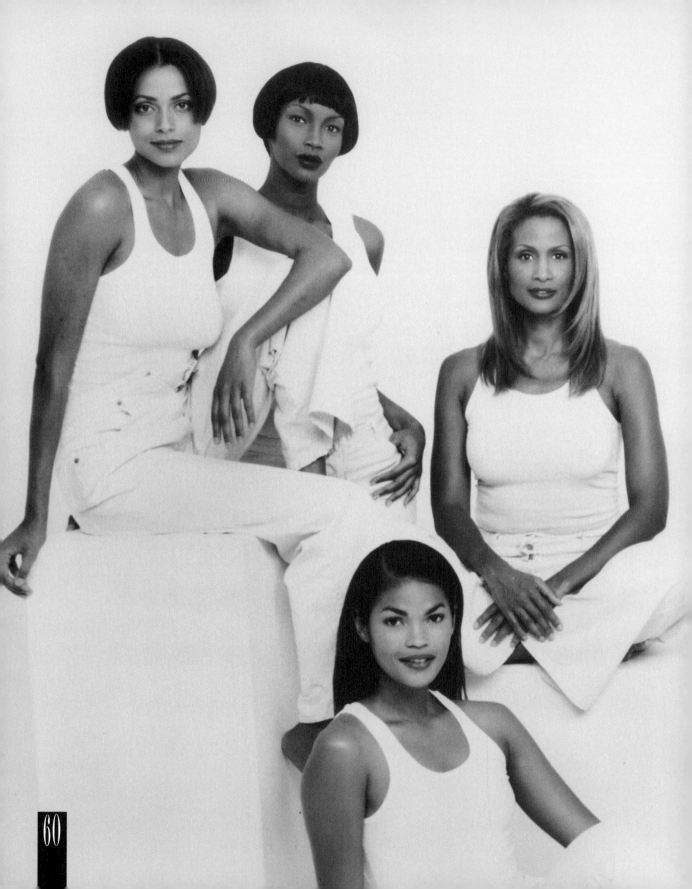

brighter—without looking overdone. Our darker, color-enriched skin is, in fact, one of the most versatile backgrounds for all sorts of makeup color, from vibrant to subtle shades.

5. Shapely, well-groomed brows not only add character and focus but act as a frame for your entire face. If you can't arch your brows yourselves, go to a pro.

6. Before applying foundation, use a good concealer to even your skin tone. If you can't find a concealer that satisfies you, try working with a foundation one shade lighter than normal (dab it gently on darkened or discolored areas) or a gold-toned or terra-cotta cream blush or eyeshadow (these work on almost any skin tone and do the job of a concealer and highlighter). Just be sure to blend!

7. Invest in the right makeup tools—the right size brushes, sponges, powder puffs. They'll serve you in good stead for many years to come. When the tool is right, the amount of makeup applied is more likely to be right too (and to glide on more effectively). **Note:** I realize that good sable brushes can be expensive, but I also know they can last a lifetime if you keep them properly. Not only will they help your makeup go on more smoothly and evenly, but they're far gentler on your skin—something you come to appreciate once you get into your thirties and beyond.

FOUNDATION: ACHIEVING THE PERFECT BASE

Does everyone need to wear foundation? Once you're out of your teens and part of the professional world—without a doubt. Even if your skin is unusually smooth and clear, foundation acts like a primer: You need it to help everything else blend smoothly and naturally.

I also believe that foundation can serve to enhance the most positive notes and tones of your natural skin color. Contrary to most makeup advice you may receive, the best foundation color is *not* always the one that matches your skin tone exactly. I like to use different foundation shades at different times, depending on the look I want to achieve.

For women of color, four different skin tones. That means the foundation colors we use varied for each of us.

How It's Done:

How to Apply Foundation like a Pro. Before applying foundation make sure your skin is clean and cool. If you're warm and perspiring, splash your face with cold water before you begin. • Put a small amount of foundation—about the size of a nickel—in the palm of one hand. Then, using the other hand, dab it onto forehead, cheeks, the sides of the nose, and chin. Blend gently outward toward the hairline, jawline, and ears and onto the neck. For an extra-perfect finish, pat with a slightly damp sponge to set the foundation and make it extra-smooth and natural.

Sometimes, for instance, I may want to bring out the gold notes of my skin with a glowing, gold-toned foundation; at other times, when I want a more suntanned, bronzey effect, I may use a deeper and richer color.

Because one of the most common makeup application mistakes I see is applying one's foundation like a heavy, skin-concealing mask, I want to emphasize that none of the foundation shades I use ever changes or conceals my natural skin color. Instead, they merely make the most of the natural tones I already have. Your own natural, beautiful skin tone should always be apparent. If you have a tendency to err in that respect, try thinking of your foundation as being a wonderfully sheer veil; whether you choose one in liquid, cream, or powder form, it should be applied so that the warmth and beauty of your own natural skin color comes through.

The type of foundation you choose is a matter of personal preference. Liquid foundations tend to offer sheer to medium coverage; creams and pressed powders provide quite a bit more. As for whether to choose a foundation that's matte or shiny, your best bet is to consider what's currently fashionable (even the most expertly applied makeup can look jarring and "wrong" when the look is simply out of date). The fact is that fashions in beauty change: Sometimes a sophisticated matte finish looks right; at other times, our eye is attracted to the moist, youthful effect of a dewier finish. What doesn't change are the basic "rules." For example, in general, a glowing, dewier finish tends to reveal skin imperfections, while one that's matte is generally kinder to problem skin. At

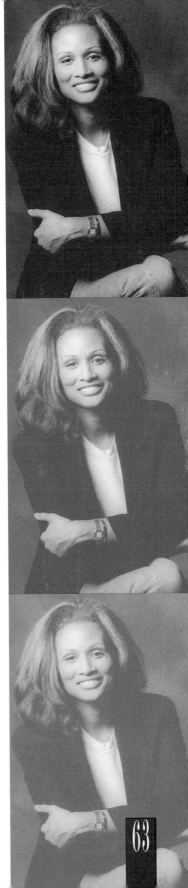

the same time, unless carefully applied a matte finish makeup on mature skin can be somewhat aging.

During most of my years as a model, I've had a hard time finding the right foundation for my particular skin tone—a situation I share with many African-American women, as well as with Asian and Latin women whose skin has deep olive or yellow undertones. The fact is that, until recently, most bases were far too pink. Even now, although so much more is available, most cosmetic collections geared to women of color offer only about twelve foundation shades—four suntan tones, four bronze tones, and four mahogany tones—simply not enough to serve ethnic women's real needs. (Not only have the selections of color been meager, but the textures themselves have been inferior—difficult to apply evenly and smoothly.)

HOW TO PICK A FOUNDATION: GETTING THE RIGHT MATCH

When you're ready to choose a new foundation, spend some time trying out the testers at the local cosmetics counter display. For the most accurate effect, try to test on bare *facial* skin only (not on your hands or arms, which are a different texture and color).

The easiest way to test a foundation is to apply a small amount of the foundation—about the size of a dime—and blend it into a "problem" or slightly discolored area, such as under the eyes or over the upper lip. Then check out the effect in daylight, not just in the artificial light of the store. If the foundation doesn't "show" and matches your neck and the surrounding skin, you've probably found

Makeup shouldn't be a mask. The warm glow of your natural skin should always come through.

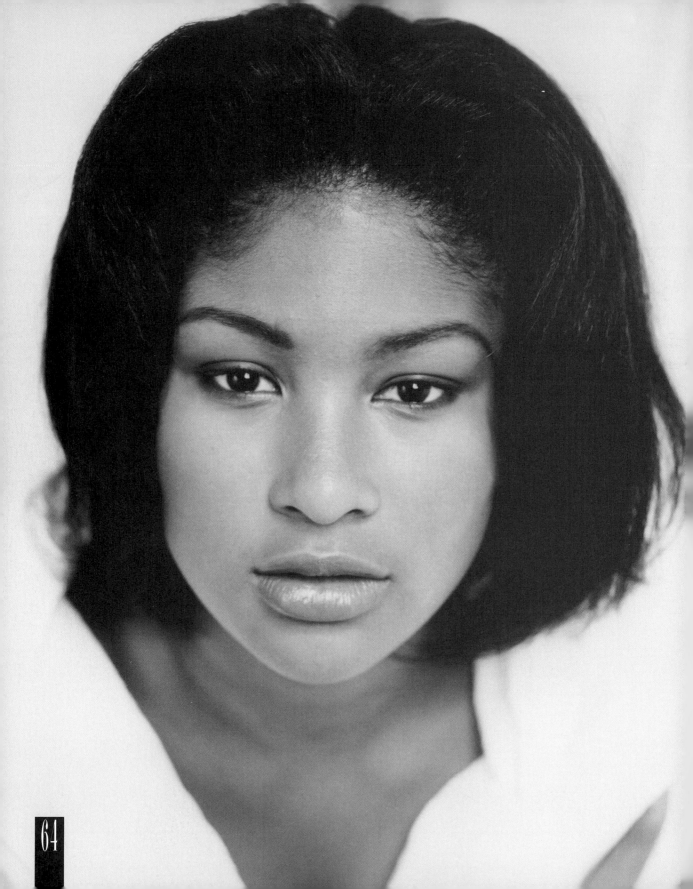

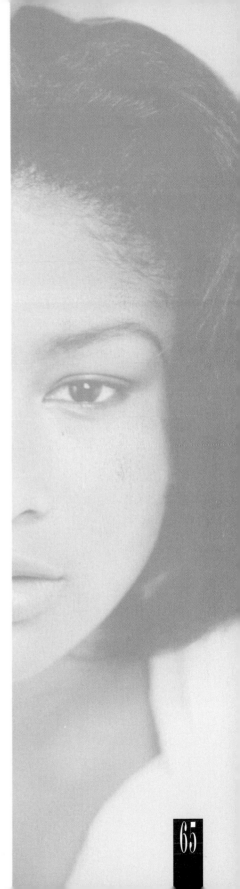

a complementary color. Keep in mind that *your foundation should either match your natural skin tone as closely as possible, or should pick up the most attractive notes or undertones in your skin*. **Tip:** When in doubt, you're probably safest going a little bit lighter than your natural skin color, as opposed to deeper, because you can always deepen and enrich the color as needed.

If, like most women, your skin tone is somewhat uneven, you may need more than one foundation—a deeper one for lighter areas, a lighter one to tone down dark spots. Using a number of colors means careful blending, of course, but it also imparts a natural look and has more staying power (that's a special plus if your skin is on the oily side). For best blending, use your fingertips or a damp makeup sponge (those little triangular sponges you can pick up at most makeup counters or pharmacies).

MAKEUP AND AGE: WHAT'S APPROPRIATE, WHAT'S NOT

Part of the fun of being a teenager is to experiment with all sorts of makeup techniques. Anansa is probably my best audience for all the tricks and professional tips I've learned during my modeling career. There's nothing we enjoy doing more on a rainy weekend afternoon than trying out some new makeup trick I've learned on a shoot, or a wonderful new shade of nail polish that one of us has picked

Anansa has become a pro at enhancing her eyes and lips without it being too much.

up. With that said, I still believe that teens look best with makeup that's applied as lightly and naturally as possible. You should never be able to notice the makeup—only the effect! I also want to caution young women about falling into the trap of spending a fortune on expensive cosmetics. At your age, a good inexpensive brand of makeup is probably your best choice.

As you move from your twenties into your thirties, possibly juggling work and family to a greater degree, it's probably a good idea to try to hone and simplify your approach to makeup. Achieving a daytime makeup that's no fuss, fairly natural, and easy to do should be high on your list. Save the experimenting and special effects for evening when you have the time to do them carefully (and then go all-out in a big way!).

Tip: If your skin is on the oily side, use a soft sponge not only to apply your foundation, but also to blot. After you've applied your foundation, wait a few minutes and check for oily spots; then blot and retouch.

What if you haven't worn much makeup in your teens and twenties, though? Chances are, you may find that as you enter your thirties, your skin may start to look a little dull and uneven in tone. This is the age when your looks may truly benefit from wearing a good foundation. Remember, if you can't find the shade you want at the cosmetics counter you can always mix and blend your own, combining earth tones, yellows, roses, golden taupes, suntanned bronzes, hennas—until you've gotten exactly the right effect. The best way to apply it: Mix it with a little moisturizer to increase the sheerness, then pat it gently under the eyes to cover dark circles, down the sides of the nose and around the mouth and cheeks, then smooth it gently over the entire face.

Another thing to remember is that the color of African-American skin can sometimes change ever so slightly, occasionally deepening and lightening as the seasons change or, sometimes, as it matures. That means that tried-and-true foundation color may need to change from season to season, or as you enter your fifties or sixties. Plus, if your skin has also gotten drier (also common as you mature), consider switching to a cream foundation. Because cream bases contain oil, they tend to be somewhat moister—a definite plus for dry skin of any color, any age.

CONCEALERS

Perhaps *the* key essential of a beautifully made-up face (but one that doesn't look made-up) is a smooth and even skin tone. This becomes our clean canvas—the

Tip:
Does Deeper-toned, More Color-enriched Skin Need "Special" Makeup? In a word, yes. It used to be that foundations and powders made for amber or cafe-au-lait-toned skins contained ingredients that turned richer, deeper skin colors an unattractive gray. Others had dark fillers (like umber) that gave darker skin an unnaturally red or yellow cast. For the most part, though, these problems have been corrected, as more companies are offering formulas designed specifically to react positively with color-enriched skin. Read labels carefully, choosing makeup with only the smallest amounts of titanium dioxide (a white pigment that often causes makeup to change color or turn chalky on color-enriched skin) or with a new translucent version or none at all.

starting point for everything else that goes on top. Although few of us have perfectly even skin tones, because of the natural variations in the pigmentation of deeper-toned skin (remember, even a simple scratch can cause the affected area of your skin to become darker—or sometimes lighter—than the rest) our foundations are often called upon to conceal as well as to provide a smooth finish for the rest of our makeup. The most common areas for dark spots or discolorations are around the lips and the chin.

This is where the use of a good concealer comes in—it's one of our most important makeup essentials. Use a concealer to accent the bridge of your nose or to remove shadows (for example, use a concealer one shade lighter than your foundation under the eyes, in the corners of the mouth, or on deep laugh lines).

When applying concealer, begin by imagining your face as a totally blank canvas. Then carefully smooth it on any shadows, darkened or on discolored areas that mar a matte, flat impression. Blend carefully to match your natural skin tone, being sure not to pull or tug at the skin.

Professional makeup artists have dozens of special tricks of the trade when it comes to evening-out skin tone and "priming" it for the rest of your makeup. One makeup artist I know suggests using a makeup slightly deeper in color; another likes using a lighter color stick; a third recommends using a golden tone to blend unevenness. And somehow they all work, beautifully! Here are the details:

• **Option 1:** Start with a foundation that's slightly richer in color than your natural skin tone. This is applied all over the face—over the eyelids, even over lips, with a damp makeup sponge (to give the foundation sheerness and more "slip"). Then it's dabbed a second time for spot applications or to blend in on any still-dark areas or shadows.

• **Option 2:** This method uses a color stick to subtly lighten the darker patches that so many of us have underneath the eyes and around the nose and lip area with the aim of getting the skin tone totally even. After that, a light translucent powder is brushed on for a smooth texture and to "set" the face. Or use a powder puff—pat on, then brush off excess for a nice, natural appearance.

• **Option 3:** This third technique substitutes gold-colored cream shadow or blush for a conventional concealer (a trick I picked up from makeup whiz Joey Mills) to give the skin a warm and natural glow. Since women of color often have yellow, orange, bronze, cordovan, or burgundy undertones to their skin, they should choose concealer color accordingly: a golden cream eyeshadow or blush if their skin is light, a medium to deep terra cotta if their skin is richer in color. Apply it under foundation to "erase" lined or discolored areas under the eyes, at the sides of the nose, in forehead furrows along laugh lines and in the nasal labial folds that run from the sides of the nose to the mouth. Then apply it over the foundation to highlight the tops of the cheekbones, the outer brow bone, the center of the eyelids, and down the center of the nose. After adding blush, dust with deep translucent powder. Blend well.

As you apply your makeup, stand back every once in a while and look at your reflection in the mirror to check whether your makeup looks natural and attractive, and whether lines of demarcation show. It's only when your skin color is totally even that you apply contour, additional highlighter, or blush. But the real secret of good makeup always comes back to that smooth and even foundation, so don't rush this step.

ESSENTIAL TOOLS

One of my basic rules is about makeup tools. How many of us spend hundreds of dollars on eyeshadows, blushers, and lip colors, on highlighters and foundations, and then apply them with old or dirty powder puffs, with cheap brushes that smear, streak, or tug at the skin, or are just not made to do the job for which they were intended? Here's what you *should* have on hand:

An Assortment of Powder Puffs. A clean powder puff is an essential. So many women don't realize that the powder puffs they use should be changed at least every three months (these come three in a pack at most discount drug stores, and there's no reason not to buy a bunch). I personally like smaller ones so that I can angle them more easily, but any size is just fine. As for the powder puffs that come in pressed powder compacts, remember that once you pat them on your skin and place them face down back into the powder, they soon become slick and coated with

FINDING YOUR "ISLANDS OF QUIET"

Some days it can be particularly hard to balance your personal and professional lives. Family pressures, school and work may make you feel like you're walking a tightrope. I try to find "islands of quiet" in the course of my day to calm and center myself. Here's a quick deep-breathing and relaxing technique that I like to do. (Remember, it's important to nurture yourself, as well as others: When you're tense and tired, even the most skillfully applied makeup is not going to be able to make a difference.)

First, relax your body, unfolding your arms and legs. Next, breathe in deeply and slowly, eyes gently (not tightly) closed. Focus on your breath, feeling and "seeing" with what is sometimes called your third eye (by that I mean your psyche, your soul, your innate intuition). Concentrate on your breath coursing through your body, going into your nostrils, your lungs, replenishing your limbs with calmness. Relax...and in just a short time—thirty seconds is all you need—you can feel yourself rejuvenated and ready to go, mind, body and soul.

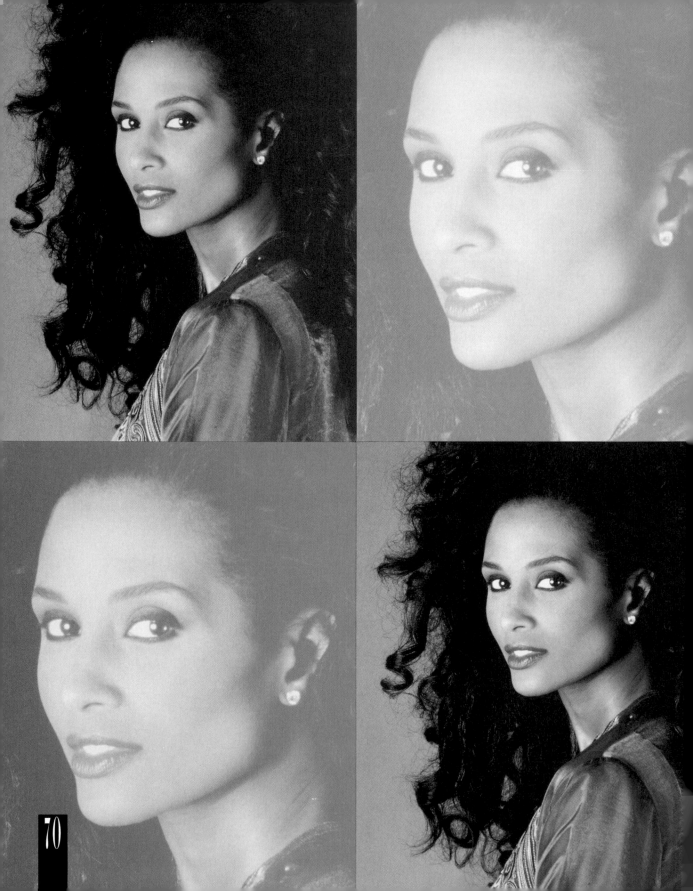

facial oil, and don't pick up the powder well anymore. To eliminate the problem, put them back face *up*. And change them every so often, because they can pick up bacteria. (Most models, by the way, prefer their powder puffs clean, but old. As with shoes, they just seem to feel better after a few weeks once you've gotten them "broken in.")

Sponges. To apply foundation, cream blush, or translucent powder, purchase some good, small triangular or wedge-shaped makeup sponges (some of these are made of silk, but any kind will do). They allow makeup to go on lightly and easily. Dampen them with water when you apply your base for the smoothest finish and to eliminate lines of demarcation. **Note:** Water can be wonderful—your best beauty aid! Try dampening powdered eyeshadow or blusher to intensify color. Also "misting" (not spraying) your face with a light, fine mist after putting on makeup can give it a special "dewy" look and help makeup stay fresh-looking. An alternative to sponges: cotton swabs to apply foundation a little at a time (also eye color or blush). It's easy...and economical.

Invest in Some Good-quality Makeup Brushes. About $100 should buy you a variety of brushes that will last for many years. If you put your money in good things, they'll pay off for you in performance.

Here's a sampling of what you should own:

• A large, full sable brush for face powder and one with a beveled edge for contour color (or try squirrel brushes, they're even softer). When you use these brushes, always flick off excess powder before sliding color across your face.

• A flat, soft blush brush (harder, stiffer brushes are meant for more direct shadowing). The brush that usually comes with blusher is generally much too small and too stiff (which means it can actually damage the fine skin around your eyes).

• A fine short angled brush for eyebrows or eyeliner, or any other strong, heavy detail. The best eyeshadow brushes are semi-stiff, for better placement (if you use a too-soft brush, the shadow will just disperse everywhere).

The right tools are essential for makeup that's this precise, this strong.

71

• A dual-purpose tapered lip brush that can outline and shape, as well as fill in with color.

• A fine-tipped shading brush made of natural hair, for eye color.

OTHER ESSENTIAL TOOLS

A flat, straight (not curved) mascara wand; pointed-tip tweezers; and cuticle scissors (to also use for brow hairs that are extremely long); an eyebrow brush; an eyelash comb; and an eyelash curler.

In order to make your daily beauty routine as efficient as possible, I also recommend that you keep your makeup neatly organized and accessible—brushes in one container, day makeup in another, evening special effects in another. If you keep things organized this way, you'll never (well, almost never) find yourself scrambling around for a makeup pencil sharpener, a clean tweezer, or the right blush. I personally like to keep my makeup in pretty little covered baskets—brushes in one, eyeshadows in another, lip colors in still another. Anansa loves those clear Lucite or Plexiglas holders, and I must admit I admire the way she organizes them. She seldom has trouble finding anything—it's all there right at her fingertips.

In addition to the practical benefits of organization, I also believe that attractive makeup containers have a lot to do with the simple feminine pleasure of the beauty ritual itself. Just the sight of your fragrance bottles and your beautifully packaged makeup

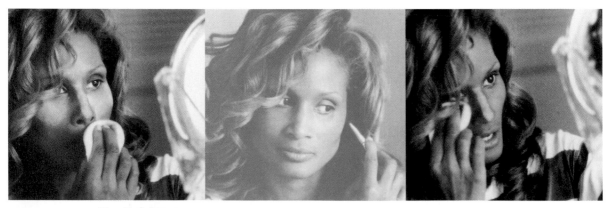

It's a ritual: doing my makeup in the natural light available at my home.

set out in elegant containers of your choice can go a long way to helping you enjoy caring for yourself. I even find that there's a special sense of luxury in owning beautifully silky makeup brushes, in taking an elegant makeup compact from your purse, or in holding a lipstick that's encased in sleek silver, elegant sapphire-blue, or sophisticated black and gold. Once again, the elegance and appeal of your makeup tools not only add to the charm of the beauty ritual but make a psychological difference in the way you feel about your looks. For instance, I carry a pretty heart-shaped, emerald-green compact in my bag (for emergency repairs) that gives me a rush of pleasure every time I use it and reinforces the positive feelings I have about taking good care of myself. It comes down to this: Because it's pretty, it can help you feel pretty, too.

Good lighting is yet another consideration. I always try to put on my makeup in the same light in which I'm going to be seen. For example, I try to

TIP

Two-minute makeup

How Long Does It Take You to Put on Your Makeup? Fifteen minutes? Twenty? That's about average, I'd say. (Although for evening and for very special occasions, some women, myself included, may spend as much as an hour!) But when I'm in a hurry I do what I call my "two-minute special."

◆

Here's how: First, dab foundation where there's an immediate need. Then take the most beautiful brown eyeshadow you own (not too strong and not too light) and stroke it on your eyelids and along the sides of your nose; blend. Add a dab of color to your brow bone and cheeks. Brush your eyebrows, filling in with pencil if needed. If you've still got a few minutes to spare, add a little brown liner under your eyes, and a fast flash of black mascara. To finish, put on a little lipstick right out of the tube—and you're out the door.

◆

apply my daytime makeup in natural light (sometimes I even move everything right near a bright window rather than putting on my makeup in the bathroom). If that's not possible, try not to put your makeup on under an overhead light, which can cast ugly and distorting shadows.

ABOUT USING COLOR

The makeup colors you'll be using most often will depend to a certain degree on what's in fashion, although not exclusively. While there will always be seasonal changes with new looks, new colors, and new textures, there will also always be those basic, unchanging guidelines that tell us how to adapt those seasonal changes to what's most suitable for us.

Because there is such a wide range of color options from which to choose, from blue-black plums to palest pink, the concept to remember is that ethnic women can wear *any* makeup color successfully, *if* we know how.

That know-how is usually dependent on three things: the sheerness of the color (sheerer is better); its tone (there are many different shades of red or shades of pink, one of which will probably work for you); and the degree of its intensity (try blending a hard-to-wear or too-bright color to an almost-nothing wash—you'll be surprised at how well it works).

Does this mean that ebony-skinned women can wear paled-out makeup shades, paler than their skin? Absolutely. I've already pointed out that pale nails look fabulous on chocolate-brown skin; so do nude lips, as long as the lip color you choose has a sheer appearance and isn't chalky. Another way to get a lightened look when these colors are popular: Try burnishing a deeper-toned lip color (like a deep berry or cordovan shade) with a gold or pink highlighter.

I personally prefer a makeup palette of earth tones and neutrals. While you initially

I've picked up many new ideas from the pros.

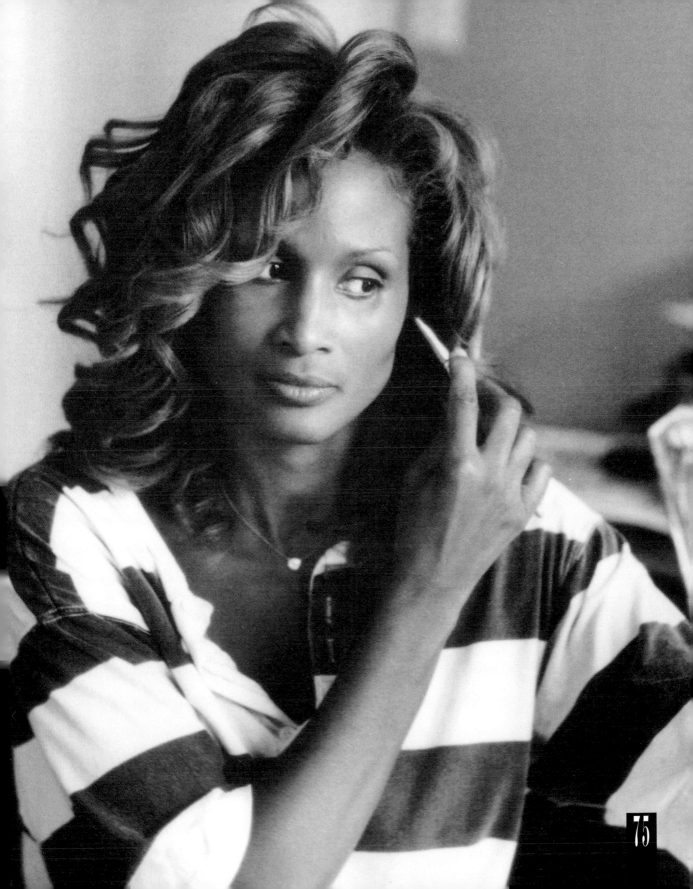

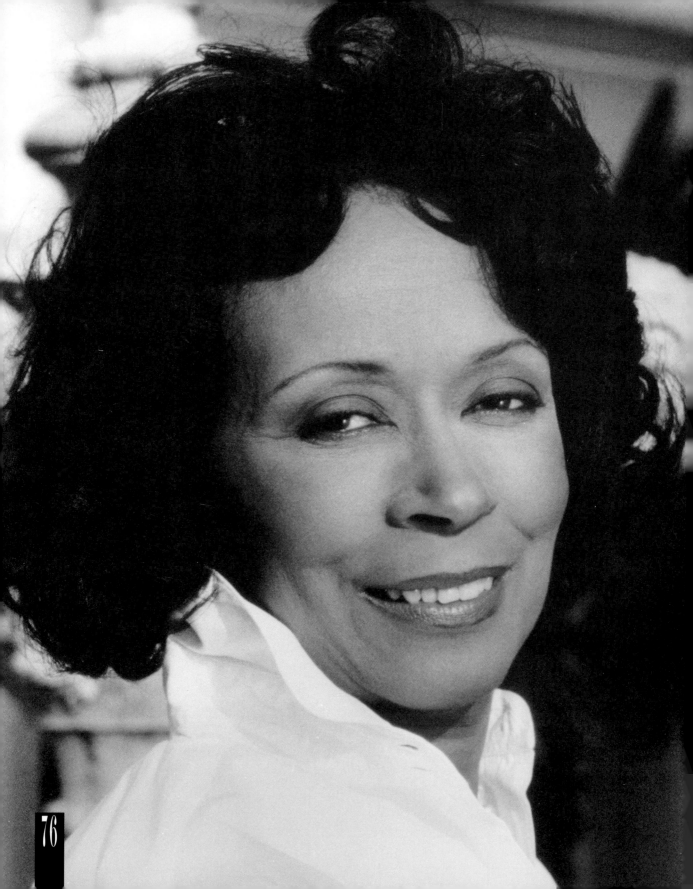

may think neutrals sound dull, think instead of rich charcoal browns, creamy taupes, and tawny russets and oranges, to name just a few. Or browns with a hint of rose or yellow in them—these can be especially soft and flattering.

The fact is that earth tones *always* work (sometimes I think Anansa and I are always looking for just the right brown or just the right taupe or a special plum for a smoky eye). I probably have at least thirty different variations in my makeup drawer right now (although somehow I never seem able to find exactly the shade of olive-green that I want!).

I strongly recommend collecting neutrals, all of which look wonderful enhanced with highlighters of gold, peach, or even pale violet, shades I also suggest you try. If your own skin tone is on the coffee-brown side, I recommend experimenting with burgundy, deep berry tones, and mauves, or with softer fuchsias and bittersweet browns. Honey tones are also a good neutral choice for beautiful, deep-brown skin. As for eyeliner, I prefer browns and brown-blacks, but navy can also work, especially on skin that's deep, rich, and lusciously brown.

Because there are so many flattering warm colors that we can wear (rusts and russets and beautiful plums) there is simply no excuse for not finding colors that work—and work well—for your own particular skin tone. That doesn't mean that anything goes, that you should run right out and buy a cherry-red blush and use it like there's no tomorrow (if you do, though, powder over it with translucent powder to make it very soft and subtle, and it should work just fine). But it does mean that there is plenty from which to choose.

In addition, knowing *how* to work with color is also a factor. One

Older women are sometimes afraid that deep colors won't be flattering. My mom proves them wrong. These earth tones are great.

of my favorite makeup artists pointed out to me that we beautiful brown goddesses can wear almost any makeup color *precisely because* we have so much rich-looking brown color in our skin. Even a screaming red is automatically softened into a far more wearable shade once it's applied to our brown base. The fact is that it's every makeup artist's dream to mix and blend beautiful color—vivid, vibrant, subtle—on beautiful skin colors like ours.

TRANSLUCENT POWDER

Before applying blusher, I like to whisk loose translucent powder all over my face (except my eyelids) with a large, soft, sable brush. This sets my makeup so that no shadings show, and also helps it last longer. How this works: When you apply the powder, you're removing excess surface oils, but leaving color. Since it's the oils that cause the foundation to shift and move, your foundation will last longer. If your skin is oily, this becomes a particularly crucial step—the oilier your skin is, the more quickly it absorbs or "eats up" makeup.

In addition, because the powder is translucent, while it doesn't add color, it does "fill in" skin imperfections, refining the skin's appearance by adding that elusive element called "finish." Whether or not you notice the difference this step makes, other people assuredly will. **Note:** Even though these powders are translucent, they're not transparent—no powder is. This means it comes in colors, usually three or four, labeled light, medium, and dark, or something similar. Choose one in the same general color family as your foundation. When you apply, don't wipe. Try to dust on as much as possible, then keep working the brush until the powder is completely dissipated.

When you're comfortable with the technique described above, here are two special insider's tricks to try:

1. Brush a little powder under your eyes to bring extra light and reflection into your face. The more light you put under your eyes, the cleaner and clearer your face will

Vivian Bernal

Beverly Peele

Judy Lue

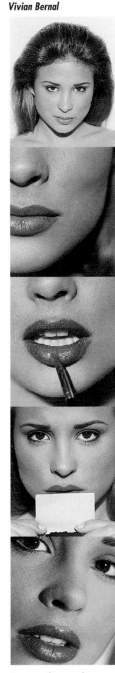

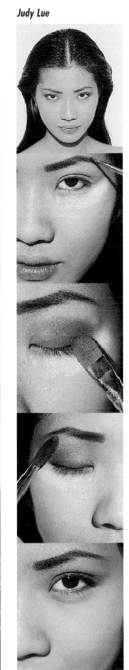

Sensuous lips coordinate with sensuous eyes for true Latin beauty.

Lighter foundation and translucent powder under the eyes plus blush highlight strong African-American cheekbones.

Rich shadows deepen exotic Asian eyes; strong brows frame eyes, face.

SHADES OF DIFFERENCE

Because of their dramatic coloring, Latin women who have deeper-toned, warm, tawny, or olive skin, and deep-brown eyes and black hair can also "take" more makeup than their fairer-skinned counterparts without looking garish or overdone. Now, this doesn't sanction a blatant or obvious hand with makeup—not at all. What it does mean is that clear and vibrant colorings—sunset orange, for example—subtly applied, can be very, very attractive. Still other options for dark-olive skin are softer, pale, but still richly colored pinks and roses. One pretty and rather unusual eye makeup combo for olive-toned skin can be a blend of soft pink and gentle gray shadows on the eyes, plus a hint of vibrant blue eyeliner (and on the lower lid, black pencil to bring out the eyes even more).

As with African-American women, Latin women shouldn't try to change—or even match—their skin tone with makeup base; rather they should use foundation to bring out and enhance the most positive natural notes and undertones of their skin. Note: When in doubt, remember that a smidgen lighter is better than deeper because you can always blend in more color as needed.

As for eyeliner, I like the effect of a warm brown or black on Latin women best.

The total
look—
sensuous,
sultry,
without
being overly
made up.

Sculptured cheekbones emphasize eyes and magnifiy chiseled features.

Creating hypnotic eyes and adding strong lip color produces a beautiful and feminine look.

appear. (Mature women who try this should dampen the area with a sponge to avoid cakiness that can emphasize wrinkles.)

2. Dab a little translucent powder around the corners of your lips. Not only will this enhance the line of your lips, but it will bring out the lip itself (and help keep your lip color from bleeding).

BLUSHER CONTOURING

Before you apply blusher and contour, your skin surface should look as smooth and as flawless as possible, but actually a little flat-looking. What blusher and contour do is bring back your face's natural highlights and planes.

Your blusher color should be in the same tone as your lip color, whether that's a coppery bronze, a peachy coral, a rose, or a magenta. Your best color will also depend on your skin tone. **Some general guidelines:** Women whose skin is lighter often look well with a beigey-gold or apricot blush. If you've got a lot of yellow in your skin, check out sienna and terra cotta shades. Women whose skin is very rich in color should veer toward auburn, fuchsia, and Indian red—all dramatic and terrific. Just keep in mind that cosmetic companies sometimes get rather fanciful and lyrical when it comes to naming their products. The label "fuchsia" printed on the cosmetic package is no assurance that it's going to be *the* fuchsia that's right for your particular skin tone. You do have to test on your own skin through trial and error. Use a clean tester or cotton ball

---

...SHADES OF DIFFERENCE

Another way: Try a little black eyeshadow, carefully smudged, instead of liner—it's a look that's a little more subtle. On lips: anything goes from a sheer, no-color gloss to a wonderful, passionate red-red!

Asian women's coloring can range from pale ivory to yellow beige. But because the latter can sometimes go sallow, it's often difficult for Asian women to find foundation that enhances their skin tone. A solution is to mix two different foundation colors (after all, no skin, whatever its color, is the same all over). You might choose one shade lighter and one darker than your own complexion and then dot it on the face following the natural lights and shadows, and blending it to create different notes of color—your own custom base. For example, you might choose foundation with a little yellow in it, another with more pronounced red, then mix them together with a little moisturizer and some water, using your hand as a palette; then see if you like the effect.

Although there are no set rules, in general a good technique for yellow beige or sallow skin is to look for warm shades, whether pale or bright. Cool colors, like blue or green, tend to overemphasize the yellow in the skin.

83

and apply to your cheekbone; then check it in daylight, not store light.

Once you've found a flattering shade, set aside the stiff little brush that comes with the blusher (if you like, you can keep it on hand for emergencies only). For daily use and the smoothest application, substitute a nice big, soft brush, about an inch to an inch and a half wide.

There are so many different guidelines as to the "best" place to apply blusher that it's no wonder that many women are confused and either misapply it or forgo it altogether. One way I recommend is to apply it in a smooth, broad stroke, brushing from the ear downward. Then use a smaller brush or a cotton ball dipped in translucent powder to blend (remember, blusher is not contour!). Another good way is the "apples of the cheeks" rule. Smile—then apply blusher on the rounded "apple" that forms. Either way, always stop cheek color two finger-widths from the nostrils. **Note:** Most pros know that it's not a good idea to use powder blush on bare skin—the texture tends to look uneven. But cream blush, dabbed on with your fingers, can work well for a casual look.

If you like, try adding a little blusher at your temples, on the bridge of your nose, or on your chin. This "sun-kissed" look can give your skin an attractive, rich tone. Just remember that it has to be subtle. Another "trick" is to sweep whatever cheek color you're using across your eye area to unify and "harmonize" the face, so the color doesn't appear spotty (this also tends to warm and soften your look). **Special note:** If you're Asian, with a decided yellow cast to your skin, a blusher with a rust or russet tone—no pinks—is probably best.

While blusher adds color, contour adds shadow and dramatic effect—and it's a very special art. I first learned about shading and contouring from the legendary makeup artist Way Bandy, who truly created and enhanced the face with expert, undetectable contouring, so that its planes picked up light in a very special way. This kind of stylized contouring is for the camera's eye only, and even when it comes to simpler contouring, unless you're fairly experienced with makeup, it's best not to try it. If you are comfortable with makeup, however, and in the mood to try some special effects, here's how:

• Most beauty experts suggest choosing a blusher in a brownish shade, slightly deeper than your skin tone, as your contour color (this is in addition to your regular blusher shade). But actually this isn't always your best choice. In fact, there's a whole range of harmonious brown shades from which to choose. A soft cinnamon-brown, for example, can be a wonderful contouring color. Or sometimes it's nice to use what I call a "burnt suntan brown" for contouring, not only on the cheeks but also over the eyebrow, or on the bridge of the nose.

• To enhance your cheekbones, contour from the ear, right under the cheekbone, brushing color into the middle of your face. Blend carefully, not in a hard line but with a soft circular motion. For a less harsh effect, and if you're confident with makeup, layer a bit of your brownish-pink blush over the contour to warm and soften it. Then use a little translucent powder once again.

• For evening or for a more sophisticated daytime makeup, you might try three or more blusher colors, all carefully blended, of course. Start on the outside of the cheekbone with a neutral shade that's slightly darker than your makeup base. Then stroke on a deeper one in the center and a brighter color, such as an apricot or a coral (not a pink), right on the apple of the cheek. Blend carefully to avoid a harsh look.

• One question I am asked frequently is, "How can I use makeup to slim down a wide nose?" First off, consider this: Just as you highlight your eyes to enhance their beauty, so you highlight your nose because you want to enhance its most positive points—not just to make it look thinner. When I apply my own makeup, for example, I like to shade the sides of my nose, not to make it look smaller but to bring out the planes of my face. With that said, here are three different strategies:

    1. Use makeup to play up your eyes. The right brow shape, in fact, can easily

minimize a broad nose. Tweeze brows into a neat, natural-looking arch, then darken with eyebrow pencil. Use shorter, light strokes with the pencil, not one hard, straight line. Then groom with an eyeshadow brush.

2. Expertise with eyeshadow can widen the eye area and thereby create the illusion of narrowing the nose. Color and contour your entire eye area using at least two shades of eyeshadow. Apply the darker shade on the lid (on and over the crease), extending the shadow at the outer corners. Add the lighter color on the brow bone. Blend the two shades together carefully and highlight the outer brow bone with a golden or terra cotta color corrector.

3. The simplest way—highlight your nose down the center with color corrector or translucent powder, then blend well. The highlighter picks up light to make the "slim" area stand out, so the "wide" area visually recedes.

Contouring can be an especially effective makeup technique for Asian women, helping to highlight the natural beauty of their facial planes and bone structure. **How-to:** Use any of the contouring techniques described above, but with a color a shade or two deeper and richer than your base, or a brownish powder blush. Top with blusher just across the cheekbones in a soft rose or apricot shade and blend well.

EYEBROWS

Eyebrows keep your look modern—it's as simple as that. Their length and shape are key in adding character and focus to your entire face. Plus, as is often noted, eyebrows act as a "frame." Just imagine how blank and bland a face would be without eyebrows, and you'll realize what an important beauty asset a beautifully shaped brow can be.

The most common mistakes that women make in making up their brows are (a) not elongating the eyebrow enough and (b) creating brows that are either too false, too strong-looking, or just uninteresting (a third mistake is to ignore them entirely). But while fashions in brow styles change—from pencil-thin and stylized in the 1930's to full and natural looking in the 1980's, and back to thinner, arched brows in the 1990's—the fact is that extremes of either style are not going to suit the day-to-day lives of most women. By all means, if you're in a trendy field, experiment with thinner brows or an unusual arch, if you have the time and know-how. But know that while thinner brows tend to open the eye area, they also require more maintenance. If you don't have a lot of time to spend on beauty routines, your best bet is to clean up stray hairs under your arch and perhaps between the eyebrows if needed. A simple, clean, groomed arch—slightly thinner and more refined when that look is current, slightly fuller when it's not—is probably most women's best bet.

Brow-shaping

How-to's. Check your brows at night before you go to bed, to take care of touch-ups and to remove stray hairs (that way, you avoid having to tweeze right before you put on makeup in the morning, when redness may show through and when makeup may clog newly opened pores). In general, the line of your eyebrows should follow your bone structure. Always tweeze from underneath. To determine where tweezing should start, there's a little trick I always use that can help: Take a pencil and use it to connect your right nostril and your inner eye corner. To determine where the brows should end, slide the pencil to the outer corner of your eye. If short, fill in with pencil in light, feathery strokes. Repeat on the other side.

EYES

Three Basic Makeups: 1. If you're in your teens (or simply not accustomed to wearing much eye makeup), approach eye makeup gradually. One good way to start is by curling your lashes with an eyelash curler. You'll be amazed at how that little lift helps expose so much more of the whites of the eyes and can make such a difference. **How to:** Simply slip the curler in place while holding your eye about three-quarters closed (you won't be able to curl your eyelashes that well with your eyes open because,

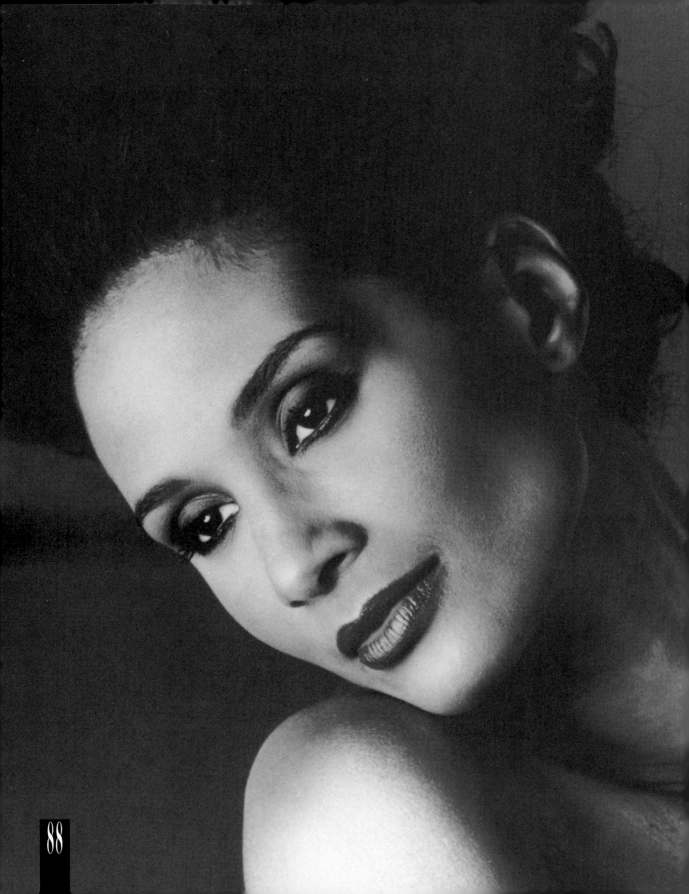

for best results, the curler should be held closely and securely at the eyelash base). Then, keeping your eye partially closed, squeeze the curler, holding for five or ten seconds. Release slowly so the lashes don't stick to the rubberized edge and pull out (after all, while lashes grow back, they do so very slowly!). Repeat twice and remove gently. Then apply your mascara before the curl droops. When you apply mascara, apply on both upper and lower lashes, concentrating on the outer corners, then comb with an eyelash comb so that each lash is separate. Repeat on the other eye.

After curling and adding mascara, apply some sheer, almost no-color gloss on your lips—and that's all the "makeup" you should need on a casual, daily basis.

2. The next level of eye makeup expertise is the addition of a single shadow in one of the all-purpose neutrals I mentioned earlier, such as a warm, tawny taupe, a beautiful russet, or a rich plum. Keep in mind that for daytime makeup, eyeshadows should be matte, as opposed to glittery, shiny, or iridescent, which should be saved for evening looks only. Apply with a sable brush, stroking across the eyelid, blending upward.

That simple touch of shadow should provide enough definition, and enough color for most occasions. For a little more finish: Add highlighter in a color slightly lighter than your skin tone, under the brow bone. Pretty choices: How about peach...or gold? And plenty of mascara (always the last step). Comb through to separate lashes.

3. A more dramatic look that consistently works well on women of color is the black-rimmed, smoky "kohl" eye, which is so reminiscent of Egyptian mysteries and beauty. Line the eye on the upper lid and inside the lower lid close to the lash line with sooty-black kohl powder. Take care not to smudge particles on your cheeks. Shadow as before, and add highlighter and mascara. **Note:** This can be a stunning look for evening, especially with a pale, no-color mouth. Another look I love: a completely neutral eye, shadowed from lash line to brow bone in golden topaz and beige tones (this can be an especially striking contrast with a strong-colored mouth and vibrant nails).

Egyptian eyes—use smokey "kohl" shadows— for a regal look.

EYE LINER

Adding eyeliner to makeup increases the emphasis to your eyes, though it's not as theatrical a look as the kohl-lined eye. I suggest dark brown, black, or occasionally navy liner along the rim of the eye, as close to the lash line as possible. However, when using a makeup pencil to line the inside lower lid, be careful. If you draw the line too close to the nose, your eyes will look close-set—and your nose wider. **Note:** If you're not used to wearing makeup, it's best to skip lining under your eyes altogether; that way you won't have to worry about it running or smudging or be concerned about touch-ups (or you can smudge it right after you apply it so that a soft, slightly smudged look is part of the makeup).

Eye Tip:
For eyeshadow to go on smoothly and evenly, the eyelids must be clean and free of oil. Before applying, pat lids gently with a bit of matte foundation; it'll help the shadow to glide on smoothly. Always use powder eyeshadow—it's not only easier to handle, but won't melt into the lid creases. • When you're brushing on eyeshadow, remember that the most color is at the outside corner of the eye (the least is closest to your nose). When you blend, always add just a little color at a time.

MASCARA

If you look at photographs in magazines, the models' eyelashes always look perfect—each lash fine and distinct, each gently curving. One reason is that right after the mascara is brushed on, while it's still wet, it's combed through with a fine-tooth eyelash comb. But even after the mascara is applied to the lower lashes, use a slanted sponge to clean up the undereye area and get rid of any telltale smudges. Because my lashes tend to be straight, not curly, I *always* use an eyelash curler with the technique described earlier (and always before I put on mascara, not afterward).

More mascara tips: Not many women know that it's important to remove your mascara before you remove the rest of your makeup. Some people like a cotton swab with a little oil, taking care not to pull at the delicate skin around the eye. I use a non-oily eye makeup remover. And I seldom use waterproof mascara precisely because it's so hard to remove without pulling and tugging at the eye area. If I cry, my mascara runs...and I just deal with it!

ASIAN EYES

Asian eyes are just so naturally beautiful and exotic-looking, it's no wonder that all women try to create our own versions of that seductive, almond-eyed effect. The best enhancement to Asian eyes is soft, smoky shadowing and plenty of mascara to highlight and emphasize their lovely shape. I've found dark matte shadows to be most effective, either in a single color or a blended range in order to create a feeling of greater depth in the lid. Also try extending the line and shadow slightly beyond the outer corners of the eyes, to emphasize their natural shape. Blend carefully. I suggest skipping

TIP

Eyeshadow looks

Although I prefer a palette of neutral browns and earth tones when it comes to eye makeup, I do like to blend and layer these shades—some lighter, some stronger—which is how I get all sorts of new effects. Russet blending into dark gray and then into black, for example, can be a dramatic look that gives the eyes lots of depth (the nicest part is that the tones tend to look like extensions of your skin tone, instead of standing out as "eye makeup" in an overly obvious way). Another beautiful combination: a soft, fresh peach on the lid, a slightly deeper tone in the crease, extending to the outer edge of the eye in an elongated look. Pale peach visually opens the eye and brings light and reflection into that part of the face, especially if your pupils are very dark.

♦

eyeliner, which often creates too harsh a line and can tend to "close" the eyes, making them look smaller. Instead, use plenty of black mascara, especially at the outer corners of the lashes, to widen.

LIPS

Most women fall into one of two extremes. Some have twenty or thirty tubes of lipstick lying in the bottom of their makeup drawer, but all of these colors are pretty much the same. This woman likes to think she's always trying something new, but the fact is that she has very set ideas about what will and will not work for her.

Other women have, at most, two lipsticks—one red, the other some kind of orange—neither of which is all that flattering. If you recognize yourself in either of these two women, I'd like to propose a better approach: a happy medium between these extremes, plus some practical, all-important lip pointers.

Before you even think about lip color—the fun part—think about lip maintenance, something I've talked a little about earlier but want to expound on here. While dry and cracking lips are one of the first signs of aging, this condition can actually happen at any age—even in your teens—when the lips are neglected. Try not to lick your lips, especially when it's cold outside. Plus, get into the habit of carrying a little lip balm around with you—Anansa and I both do, and we slather it on whenever we remember to keep our lips moist and smooth. **Note:** If your lips are cracking, use just a touch of lip color—the thinnest gloss. Too much color while your lips are still healing will accentuate the cracks.

The next thing to know is that the effectiveness of lip color is determined in large part by the skin color over which it goes. Since many African-American women have uneven lip color (like me: my top lip is brown, my bottom one pink), you might want to use lip liner not only to line your lips but to shade in the entire lip area (a trick that also has the advantage of helping your lip color last longer). Sometimes I do this, lining and evening out the color of my lips first, then applying lipstick or sheer gloss on top; at other times, I leave my lips the way they are naturally. You can use a concealer, to prime your lips and even out the color, before lining and applying lipstick. It's entirely up to you.

Full, sexy lips, of course, have been "in" for a long time. But if you think yours are too full (if your lips are pale, by the way, they may look fuller than they really are), you can visually reduce their size by lining them with a deep-toned pencil and filling them in with color. Top with a lip color that complements your skin tone (a sienna, a terra cotta, burgundy, or cordovan). And look for sheer formulations, which are less likely to cake or turn red.

Some women tell me they feel their lips are too big only on the bottom. To visually disguise a droopy lower lip, use makeup to shade and shadow, lining your lower lip with

lip liner, then filling it in with color, but leaving the center a little bit lighter. This won't necessarily make your lips look small and thin—nor would you want it to—but it will enhance and flatter their shape, which is the main idea.

For lip liner, I tend to prefer natural brown or taupe shades. Often I find myself mixing and custom-blending a color to get exactly the shade I want. Remember, though, that when

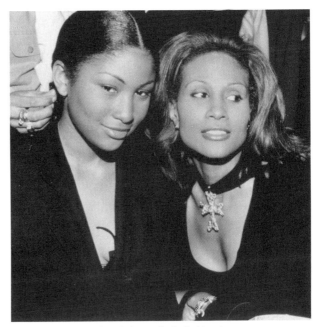

Anansa, getting a touch-up before a charity fashion show.

I talk about liner, I'm not talking about anything harsh, obvious, or stylized (that's why you should never use lipstick color as a pencil—the line is too harsh). The purpose of liner is to add definition and bring your lips into focus, something that is particularly important if your skin is on the deeper, more ebony-enriched side.

EVENING MAKEUP

Sometimes your evening makeup doesn't have to be all that different from a great daytime look. What I suggest for evening makeup and other special occasions is to strengthen your daytime makeup and that's it. What that means is to increase the amount of color you use, largely because you're going to be seen, literally, in a different (usually darker and dimmer) light, so you want your makeup to still show. (Rich, rosey reds on the lips, for instance, can be especially wonderful in candlelit restaurants or in dark, night club-like atmospheres.)

The texture of lipstick makes it suitable for many things, not only lip color. Try a plum lipstick, for instance, as a blush on your forehead and cheeks, or to contour your chin. (Tip: you can blend the color outward with your thumb to decrease the width of your chin.) Just don't use lip color on your eyes.

To compensate for the change in light, you may also want to change the colors you use, going for a slightly deeper or richer eyeshadow, or a highlighter with a hint of iridescence to suggest a shimmer. Other differences: additional contouring, a more defined lip line, adding eyeliner (liquid can be effective) if you don't usually wear it by day. Or, use a more brilliant lipstick, dramatized with a rich gloss. To highlight bareness at night, try a shimmer of iridescent powder above and below the collarbone to catch the light.

Once you know these general guidelines, keep in mind that there are exceptions. Evening makeup depends on the situation, and there are places for wonderful, more

TIP

Some good lip techniques:

1. After lining your lips and filling them in with color, smooth on a dark mahogany or russet brown lip color. Then apply a slightly lighter shade on the inside of the lip; blot; go back to the darker shade; blot again. Continue layering light on dark, so that there are many layers of color, all of which should be very long-lasting. Another way to help lipstick last longer: Outline lips first with a matte lip liner. Then apply lipstick, with a lip brush (never directly from the tube). Blot with a tissue, dust with translucent powder, then brush on another layer of color, and blot again.

♦

2. Use shadows on your lip to intensify the color and "bring it up." The same brown shadow that you use on your eyes can be rubbed into your lips, blotted, then glossed over.

♦

3. Tips on lip color: The most common mistake I find in terms of lip color is choosing a shade that isn't complementary to your skin tone—looking for immediate color that "pops" rather than for a soft and flattering shade. This often happens when lip color is the only makeup you're wearing. Unfortunately, wearing just lip color, with no makeup on your eyes or cheeks, tends to emphasize the lips disproportionately, and can throw the color harmony of the entire face out of balance.

Mind you, it's not that I don't like a good strong lip color. I do—just not alone, as the only element of color on your face. Better choices: any good, warm shade, flattering to your skin tone (as long as you're lining them first, it's hard to go wrong). To try: rich russets (rather than hard, vivid oranges), brown-based plums, soft grapey tones, and bronzes. All of these are colors that suggest softness but don't scream. And even when it's not the fashion, I always keep a red lipstick on hand, just in case; every once in a while, there's nothing more sexy or inviting than red lips! The best reds for ethnic women: I find that rich blue-reds are sexy and terrific on ebony-skinned women (you don't want the red to be too bright or there will be too much contrast between your lips and your skin tone). Women whose skin is a medium-toned coffee brown like mine might try a clear, cherry red (my best all-around red!). A true bright "Chanel" red can also be very flattering. As for brighter-skinned women with a lot of yellow in their skin, a beautiful orangey-red works especially well.

Whatever lip color you end up using, always apply it with a brush, rather than straight from the tube. A brush lets you control the color and allows for a neater, more natural look.

♦

exaggerated fantasy makeups (with sequins, with playful false eyelashes, with unusual or dramatic colors that you wouldn't normally wear). Rich smoky eyes and a gilt-edged liner, for example, can provide a strong dose of evening glamour for a gala evening out. Or lips brushed with a provocative, satiny shine, instead of a bright gloss. You might try a brilliant fuchsia eye, adding the color not only on the eyelids or brow, but also on the tops of the cheeks. Blend with a pearly silver to contour and add light. How about shadowing your eyes with black charcoal, extending the shadow out to the outer corners of the eyes for the most dramatic effect? For lips, you may want to try stronger corals than you would by day, or deep maroon reds and glistening golds.

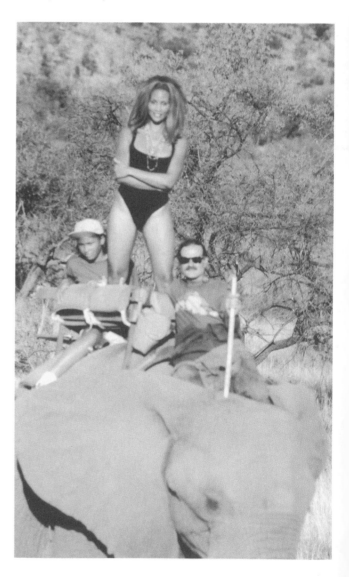

There are also circumstances where you can break all the rules and still look wonderful. Although blue and turquoise eyeshadows should generally be approached with caution by ethnic women (they can look overly artificial and exaggerated), if I were on an island vacation, on a sandy beach and dressed all in white, I certainly wouldn't hesitate to put a very heavy strip of incredible turquoise color on my eyes.

On occasions like this one in Africa, I get a kick out of trying creative and wild makeup and outfits.

BEVERLY JOHNSON

Finally, because women today have less time than ever to spend on themselves yet have never been more concerned with looking good and feeling fit (it's no accident that when I think about a good daily basic routine, I inevitably think of words like "streamlined," "simplified," and "basic"), we've become more quality conscious when it comes to makeup. The makeup you buy and wear should be able to stand up to many demands. Before you leave the cosmetics counter, ask yourself: Is the color neutral? Will it work with my skin tone? Will it fit easily in a cosmetics case or in my purse? Will it last—through lunch? And if I don't have time to change after work, will it work if I have to go directly from the office to dinner? Today's active woman imposes the same standards—of practicality and efficiency—on her beauty regime as she does on other areas of her life.

♦

PAY ATTENTION TO THE MAINTENANCE PROCESS

As a model who is being constantly photographed, I'm probably more aware than most people of the small changes in the texture of my skin and the necessity for daily upkeep. Still, for all of us, true beauty is a matter of constant maintenance and care. This means it's important to pay attention to the small changes you see in your appearance; don't let things go. If your skin seems a little dry one day, go for that moisturizing mask. If your face seems drawn with lines of tension or stress, take the time out to meditate or do yoga to smooth away those temporary worry lines, which will release as you relax and unwind. Lips especially are a special point for me—so few women realize that their lips need to be cared for. Especially as you mature, your lips may become prone to drying and cracking and may need constant moisturizing, protection, and attention.

97

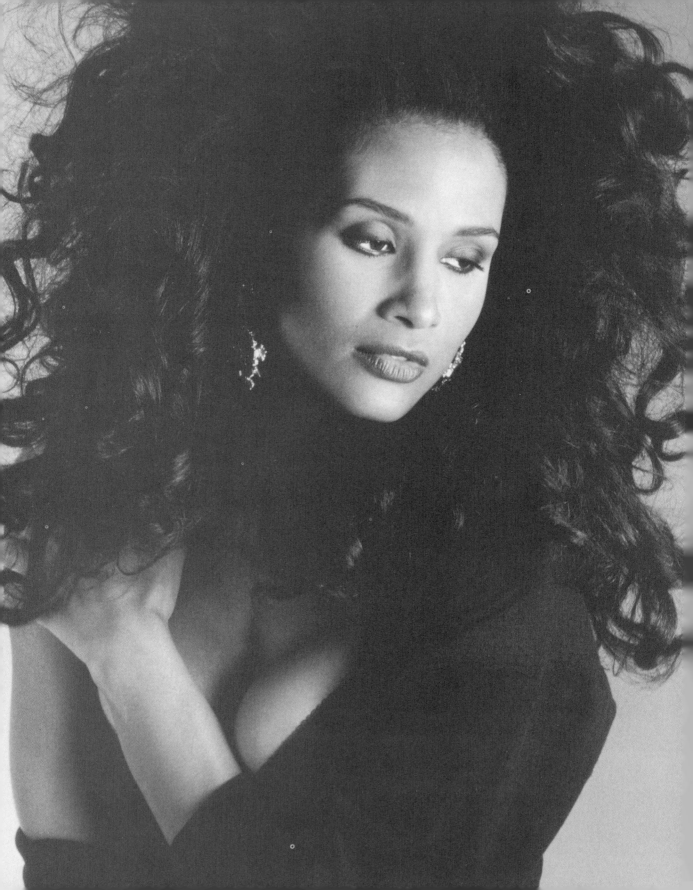

Chapter 4

True
Beauty
Hair

Super Hair: A Woman's Glory

Here's everything you need to know regarding cut, color, special care, conditioning, styling, relaxing, extensions, weaving, tools, hair buying, trends, and more.

Are we obsessed with our hair? Maybe. Healthy, beautiful hair is probably the top beauty priority for most women and we have no qualms about spending hour upon hour on our hair to make it look just the way we want it. Statistics say that, as a group, ethnic women, particularly African-American women, do tend to spend more time, more effort, and more money on our hair than our Caucasian counterparts. Whether it's a matter of taking the time to sit under a dryer for an hour and a half, or fussing with curlers, hot rollers, and straightening irons, we do it. After all, throughout history, hair has been heralded as a woman's crowning glory—and that's never been more true than it is today.

Perhaps it all goes back to centuries-old African traditions, when women spent hours patiently and painstakingly adorning their hair with colored beads and metal ornaments, with feathers and clay coloring, and of course braiding and weaving their hair into intricate masterpieces. What I do know is that when my hair looks good, I feel complete and at my best. You probably do, too.

Because of the versatile texture of African-American hair, we can literally wear it more ways than any other racial group. Its tightly curled, interlocking texture (experts say it includes a flattened twist about every half inch in each single strand) is what enables us to indulge not only in pulled-back chignons, chin-length, layered bobs, and spiky bangs, but in all sorts of sculptured styles, in braids, cornrows, Nubian twists and dreadlocks, and glamorous beaded and thread-plaited styles. One stylist I know said that it's precisely because of its versatility that it's so wonderful to work with African-American hair. With the right styling tools, you can make any beautiful hairstyle imaginable.

While the texture and wave pattern of African-American hair may vary, most of us—70 to 90 percent, in fact—resort to chemical processing such as relaxers to soften, smooth, and straighten our hair in order to increase its pliability and versatility (not, as so many people erroneously believe, to imitate the properties of Caucasian hair!). But while relaxing does make our hair easier to handle, the fact is that it also weakens and dries it, making it more prone to damage and breakage.

Maybe it's contradictory, but while our hair is strong (for example, it certainly can be resistant to coloring techniques, and requires hot combs and strong chemical solutions to break down its bond), it's also inherently fragile. Even without the abuse it takes from an often excessive use of relaxers and straightening tools, if not treated kindly it can split and break. The key to achieving the great hair that we all want, then, is knowing that our hair is *sensitive* and treating it accordingly. Daily brushing and combing, for instance, should be done as gently as possible to avoid harmful friction; be sure to lift or fluff your hair only when it's slightly damp and easier to comb. In addition, plenty of regular conditioning, both remedial and preventive, is probably the single most important element of care needed to keep your hair healthy and in good shape.

Conditioning means additional moisture, in the form of moisturizing shampoos and the frequent use of heavy-duty conditioners. Since our hair can be damaged easily by the wrong products, I've always enjoyed experimenting with natural hair conditioners to combat the effects of the ever-changing hairstyles that are a constant part of modeling. One I always advocate: mayonnaise, which can be one of the best deep-conditioning treatments you can find. If you compare the labels, you'll see that mayonnaise contains many of the same ingredients as commercial conditioners: protein and acid (in the form of eggs and vinegar) and lots and lots of oil. **How to:** Just smooth it on slightly (not soaking) wet hair, cover with a plastic shower cap, sit under the dryer for fifteen minutes, then shampoo at least two or three times to get all the mayonnaise out.

Sleeping on a satin pillowcase at night is also a good idea to help reduce stress on the hair (it also helps your hair stay cleaner and keeps it from getting "smashed").

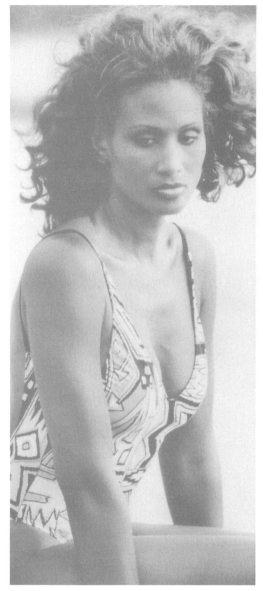

Make sure your hair always has conditioner on it when you go to the beach; it'll help prevent sun damage and hair breakage.

Why does our hair break so easily? One reason is that every twist in African-American hair represents a potential stress point. That means the curlier your hair, the more prone it is to breakage. Black hair is also prone to a condition in which the individual hairs catch on each other, which causes fragmentation when they're rubbed. Still another cause of breakage can be the traction caused by cornrows left in too long. All of these factors—plus the effects of chemical processing (and sometimes coloring as well), and despite the availability of many more quality hair-care products than ever before—means that our hair simply must be handled with *tender loving care* to avoid breakage and bring out its beauty.

KNOWING YOUR HAIR-CARE BASICS

Let's start with the basic characteristics that make our hair unique. Is it the texture? The chemistry? The range of colors?

Facts to Know. Although there certainly are exceptions, African-American hair is usually coarser in texture, tighter in curl pattern, and more delicate inherently, as well as more vulnerable to damage from chemical treatments. Because of our multicultural heritage, though, remember that there really isn't any one typical "type" of African-American hair. Its texture can vary from fine to medium to coarse; its curl pattern from straight to softly wavy to excessively tight; its colors from blonde, to red, to all sorts of browns, to black.

One myth I often hear repeated again and again about our hair is that it doesn't "grow." In fact, African-American hair grows just as quickly (or as slowly, depending on your point of view) as Caucasian hair does—about one-quarter to one-half inch per month, which is about six inches a year. Black hair only *seems* to grow slowly, partly because hair growth is just not as noticeable on tightly curled hair, and partly because of the amount of hair breakage to which we're prone. So to stay in good shape, your hair does require frequent trims—about every six weeks is a good guideline. As you grow older though, hair *does* grow at a slower rate, so it's wise to consider that before cutting your hair super-short.

There is no chemical difference in the makeup of African-American hair in comparison with any other hair type. It has a cuticle (the outer layer), a cortex (the middle layer, composed primarily of keratin and moisture, plus melanin, which gives our hair its color), and a medulla (the center of the hair shaft). All these parts are identical to those of Caucasian hair. What is different is our wave and bonding pattern. (Bonding relates to the structure of the hair: the tighter the bond, the curlier the hair.)

Although our hair color can vary from a very light, sandy blonde to dark black, in general, ethnic women do tend to have rich-brown complexions and deep-brown hair. Yet there are many different tonal qualities to African-American hair—from medium browns and reddish mahogany to darkest blue-black. Latin women's hair ranges in color from medium brown to black; Native American and women of Indian descent usually have pure black hair. In Asian women, hair color ranges from very dark glossy browns to pure blue-black, with 90 percent falling into the black range.

Around 90 percent of Asian women have straight, thick, shiny dark-brown or black hair, which calls for its own unique beauty and care considerations. The key difference: the cuticle—that is, the outermost layer of hair—is exceptionally compact on the surface. This tighter surface layer not only adds more light reflection, which accounts for the slick, shiny look of Asian hair, but also makes it less prone to damage. On the downside, the compactness of Asian hair can make it more resistant to setting techniques, and in some cases, though not all, impede the penetration of chemicals, such as perms or color. That's why, despite its beauty, many stylists find that Asian hair is the hardest to work with since in general it's not pliable and can tend to be coarse and spiky, especially when short.

Latin hair is similar to Asian hair. It shares its enviable thickness, shine, and a degree of coarseness. But its texture varies from straight to wavy to tightly curled—about 75 percent of Latin women do have some kind of curl or wave movement in the hair. For the most part, Latin hair is great—it's lush and wavy, and hair stylists say it's fairly easy to work with. However, some Latin women complain that their hair can be so thick and curly that it becomes unmanageable. And, like Asian hair, the compact cuticle of Latin hair can make it somewhat difficult to penetrate, which means it can be resistant to straightening and coloring. In coloring Latin hair, for instance, it's often difficult to remove the natural pigmentation, which is why so many Latin women who opt for coloring end up as redheads.

SHAMPOOING

Just as there is not one foundation color that suits every skin tone, so there's no such thing as one shampoo for every head of hair. Hair comes in many tones and types, just as skin does, and requires individual attention.

Asian and Latin women usually need to shampoo more frequently than

African-American women since oil buildup can be more noticeable. Depending on your hair, it can be every other day or every third day.

African-American women should shampoo their hair no more than once a week, preferably once every ten days, to avoid drying it out (once styled, our hair can be left up for a week or two—it's not "wash and wear hair"). Exceptions: models or actresses or women who spend time under hot lights or working in the outdoors should definitely shampoo more often. Another exception: after a strenuous workout in the gym. Following vigorous exercise, if your hair is drenched in perspiration, be sure to rinse it thoroughly with warm water since salty perspiration can dry out your hair.

The type of shampoo you choose is really a matter of personal preference and the texture of your hair. For instance, hair that is on the coarse side—and that usually includes Asian, Latin, and African-American hair—generally benefits from a moisturizing shampoo. **Note:** If your hair is thick, you probably won't have to shampoo as often as someone with fine hair, because the natural oils won't be as noticeable (oils tend to quickly weigh down fine hair, making it limp and lank).

In general, select a mild moisturizing shampoo that's made for your particular needs and hair type (the usual categories are dry, normal, oily, color-treated, chemically processed and damaged). Keep in mind that protein shampoos can be drying unless they're balanced with a moisturizer (an important consideration if, like most women of color, your hair has been chemically processed and is therefore on the dry side). Silk protein and milk protein shampoos and those with hydrolyzed human keratin can be particularly good because they coat the hair, giving it more flexibility and the luster it lacks naturally. **Note:** About pH: You've heard about pH-balanced shampoos over and over again. All it means is this: A low pH number—like 3 or 4—on a shampoo label just means a high acid content. This is usually a good thing for damaged hair. Since perms and chemical relaxers are highly alkaline, an acidic shampoo smoothes the

Everyone's hair has its own unique texture—wavy, straight, tightly curled. Whatever it is, learn to work with it...and, to enjoy it.

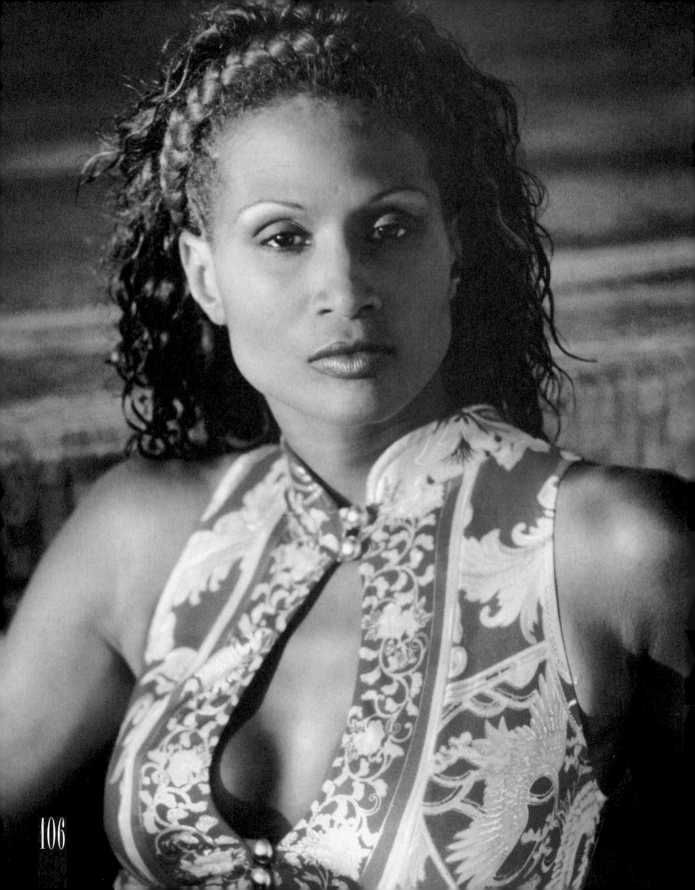

roughened hair cuticle and helps make the hair shinier, less porous, and easier to comb. A high pH number—like 9—means a high alkaline content, which is best avoided since it can leave ethnic hair overly dry and brittle. If your hair isn't particularly damaged, something in the middle, about pH 7, should be just right.

In the past, African women have traditionally used natural products like lemongrass and shea butter on their hair. Perhaps with that in mind, I have a tendency to seek out natural products as well. Shampoos that contain jojoba, a healing, soothing plant extract, which leaves my hair soft and in the most beautiful shape, are a special favorite, as are those with aloe vera or rose water. Good to try: shampoos with chamomile, nettles, or comfrey (these botanicals are natural conditioners that won't "strip" the hair). Also, most experts advise black women to steer clear of anything that contains alcohol (too drying) or balsam (not enough moisturizing benefits).

More tips for all ethnic hair types: Even if you find a shampoo that you like, it's a good idea to switch shampoos occasionally to prevent the buildup of residue that can weigh the hair down and make it limp. In a sense, your hair "gets used to" a particular shampoo and truly benefits from the switch. When you shampoo, wet your hair first, place shampoo in the palm of your hand and blend it evenly between your hands. Then apply the shampoo at the roots of the hair,

Regular conditioning, mostly with natural products, means I can wear my hair almost any way I want...as here, wrapped with a braid, the back just natural.

CONDITIONERS

Some of the best conditioners are those that you make yourself—"home remedies," I call them. One easy one that I like: watercress, rubbed directly on the scalp or put through a juicer and used as a rinse. Or thyme—just brew it as you would tea, then let it cool in the refrigerator and apply. The avocado pack, a treatment I've advocated for a long time, has always been one of my favorites, especially for dry, brittle, or damaged hair. How to: Right before shampooing, mash the pulp from a whole, ripe avocado with a teaspoon of olive oil, then store in the refrigerator in a tightly covered bowl until you're ready to use. After shampooing, section your hair, and smooth on the purée from roots to ends. Cover your head with a heat cap (or wrap your hair in plastic wrap) and sit under a hood dryer for at least twenty minutes. The heat from the dryer helps the oil from the avocado really pentrate the hair shaft and scalp. Rinse thoroughly.

For occasional dandruff, right after you shampoo and condition your hair, massage a generous amount of Sea Breeze astringent into your scalp. Let set for a minute, then rinse, and you'll find it will stop your scalp from flaking.

working it into a lather, concentrating on the scalp area. Always use the flat part of the fingers—not the nail tip—and gently massage the scalp (some people say the massage stimulates hair growth). Handle your hair carefully, especially if you've recently had a chemical treatment, but do rinse scrupulously. The reason: Treated hair can be porous and tends to hold on to dulling residue—not an attractive thought.

After shampooing, use a detangler to give your hair more "slip" and reduce the potential trauma of pulling (put a little on your palms, then apply to hair from the roots to the ends and comb through). Of course, the only comb you should use on wet hair is a wide-tooth one. After it's dry, brush your hair gently with a good brush—long, stiff bristles are best—like a Mason Pearson.

CONDITIONING

Because I have to change my hair styles so frequently, I rely on nourishing hair conditioners to keep it in good shape. In addition to the mayonnaise treatment

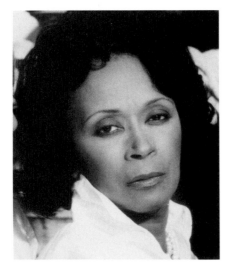

Glorious, sensual hair has no age limit. Ask my mom, Gloria.

I mentioned earlier, a warm olive oil treatment is also an effective natural conditioner for straightened hair. Heat olive oil in a saucepan (take care not to make it too hot!) and dab it on the roots of your hair with a cotton ball. Then wrap your hair in a hot towel and wait for twenty to thirty minutes. Another option is to wrap your hair in a plastic bag and sit under a dryer for twenty to thirty minutes. Shampoo out *thoroughly*. If your hair is very dry, try a few tablespoons of plain yogurt

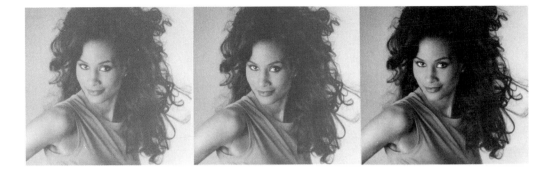

mixed with an egg. Apply the mixture to wet hair (especially the ends), wrap your hair in a hot towel or shower cap, wait fifteen to thirty minutes, then shampoo and rinse.

Whatever conditioner you decide to try, remember that regular conditioning is the *only way* to restore the appearance of chemically processed hair. Chemical processing, misuse of straightening appliances, and rough handling of the hair erodes and damages the hair cuticle. Conditioners smooth that damaged outer surface by coating the hair (they don't penetrate) and by putting back oils and proteins that chemical processing and some shampoos skim off.

In addition, since African-American hair is curly (which means it doesn't catch and reflect the light the way straight hair does), conditioning also helps flatten and smooth the cuticle of each individual hair and thereby boosts the shine.

Most experts suggest conditioning your hair once or twice a week, with either a wash-out or a leave-in conditioner. For natural, unprocessed hair, regular conditioning with a wash-out conditioner should be all that's necessary to keep your hair in good shape. For relaxed or colored hair, particularly if it's sustained some damage, or to give pliability to thick, straight, coarse hair, it's a good idea to also use a deep-conditioning treatment about once a month (apply to damp hair once you've gotten out of the shower). Either way, remember that, as with skin, your hair's needs change; what works

Even when you're wearing extensions, it's important to condition all your hair— extensions included—not just your own.

in the summer may not work in the winter. That means it's important to adjust your treatment and care accordingly.

What about other hair-controlling and replenishing products? A pomade is essentially a styling aid that adds shine, moisture, and control to your hair (use just a little at a time on the surface of African-American hair or on Latin hair that's thick, coarse, and curly). "Hairdressing" is another term you may come across. Technically, although a pomade is a form of hairdressing, the term "hairdressing" usually refers to a lighter formulation that can also be used for shine and control. "Hair polishers" and "shine creams" work the same way, helping to mold and style, while adding luster. **Note:** Be sure to keep pomades and oils away from your hairline and off your forehead since they can cause breakouts or aggravate existing acne.

A pomade is essentially a styling aid that adds shine, moisture, and control to your hair.

If you want your hair to look shinier but don't care to use anything as heavy as a pomade, try working a light hair oil into your hair after conditioning. This can add flexibility as well as sheen (and those that are made from the new water-soluble formulas don't build up or attract dust). Two good ones are Sebastian Laminates Concentrate Gel, a water-soluble, silicone-oil base that builds in body, flexibility, and shine, and Let's Jam Power Shine, which I find helps eliminate the frizzies.

Healthy Asian hair usually needs minimal conditioning; sometimes all that's necessary is a protein-based conditioner on the ends only. Once every few weeks, though, deep conditioning with a heavy-duty moisturizing cream is a good idea. **Note:** For very thick, straight hair, such as Asian hair, avoid high-alcohol gels and gels that slick or super-hold the hair. This is because when the hair is very straight, these products will create a noticeably stiff appearance and may separate the hair. The goal for this hair type should be softness, pliability, and control—but without stiffness. Use instead: leave-in conditioners and gels that give hair more control without hardness. Simply apply to damp hair, then style as usual.

Every kind of hair can benefit from a rest from straightners, permanents, and chemicals, and from extentions and weaves that can pull on the hair, causing stress and breakage. For one month each year, why not try wearing your hair washed and loosely braided, to give it a chance to revive?

BASIC STYLING TOOLS

What are the basics you'll need for everyday?

• A selection of combs—a wide-tooth comb (one with rounded tips is gentle for sensitive scalps); a comb for detangling wet hair; one with extra-wide spaces between the teeth for combing extra-curly hair

• A good brush (a Mason Pearson or a Denman, which has plastic teeth and is more like a comb)

• A vent brush, if your hair is very curly

• A good styling comb with a pick on the end

• A straightening iron for smooth styles

For styling purposes, you might want a blow dryer with a comb or vent brush attachment (and a built-in or detachable pick with which to lift, straighten, and shape the hair). Since not all African-American hair has to be pressed or relaxed, a good blow dryer and a brush, used gently, can also be used to smooth and "straighten" your hair if it isn't excessively curly. Other essentials to keep on hand: a curling iron (a large barrel for a loose curl, a small barrel for tight) and a set of rollers. Some choices: mesh rollers, used with large hair pins to avoid roller dents; sponge rollers, with the ends wrapped in Kleenex to prevent dents; and Velcro rollers, which produce smooth, shiny, bouncy results.

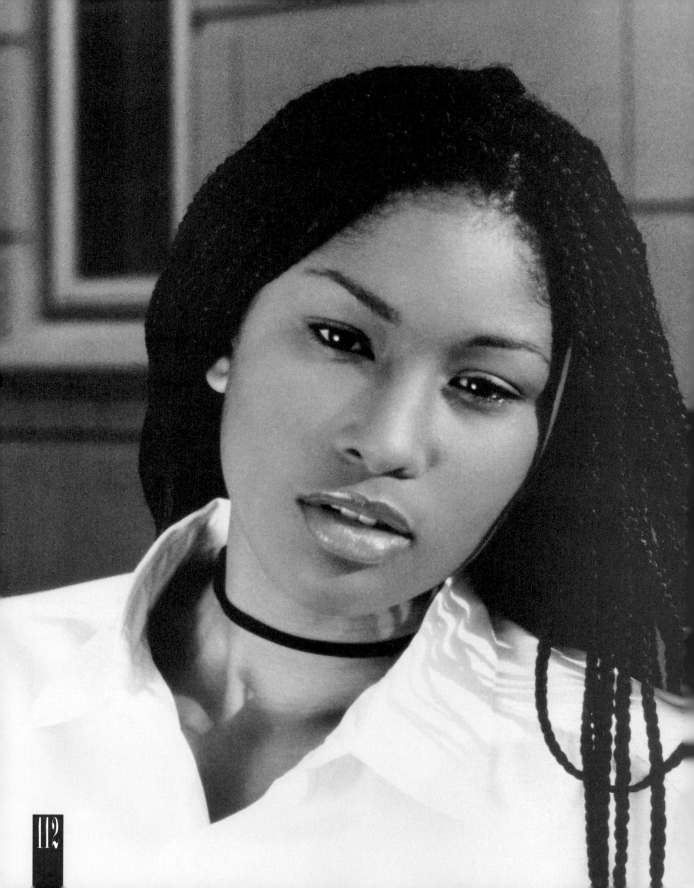

Another warm-set option that can be less damaging than curling irons or hot rollers are steam rollers. These consist of a flat plastic roller with a sponge in the center that is filled with water and salt to produce steam when heated. Hair is wrapped around the roller, covered, and left in according to the manufacturer's directions.

CURLING IRONS AND BLOW DRYERS

You've probably noticed that hair-care appliances made specifically for African-American hair (mainly electric curling irons and blow dryers) have become quite a growing market. Because our hair is thicker than Caucasian hair, conventional curling irons often don't do as good a job. Plus, when a conventional curling iron is used, the hair may absorb so much heat that the iron can take as long as twenty minutes to reheat.

Curling irons designed for African-Americans, on the other hand, are

Braids can be a timesaver in the long run because they eliminate daily use of blowers and conditioning irons—which can be hard on your hair. But frequent washing and conditioning is still a must.

TIP

Blow-drying tips for thick, straight hair (Asian, Latin)

Blow drying can help give thick, straight hair more control. Some pointers:

For short hair—blow dry and scrunch hair with fingers for more volume.

◆

For chin- to shoulder-length hair—dry using a large, round brush and turning the hair under.

◆

For long hair—blow dry and brush out. For extra oomph, when you're at a salon have your hair flat-ironed after blow drying, which is like "straightening" straight hair. It seals the cuticle, and gives it extra shine, movement, and swing.

◆

specifically made to work with our thicker hair, which requires ultra-hot temperatures to straighten or curl. Because of these higher temperatures, the surface of the barrel should be gold-plated to keep it from melting. These special curling irons also have the advantage of heating up more quickly, and of reheating within seconds during the curling process.

For best results in styling, select a curling iron with variable temperature controls, from low to ultra-hot (which most standard models don't have), since different types of hair need different settings. Even so, it's best not to use the hottest setting on your hair, and never let the heat touch your scalp.

PLAYING IT STRAIGHT: RELAXERS, PERMS, STRAIGHTENERS

Easier maintenance—it's one of the special concerns that we have about our hair, and straightening or relaxing it is probably the best way to achieve that goal. Quite simply, relaxed hair is easier to deal with. Why shouldn't we have the advantages of easy care, manageability, and more styling options that straightened hair allows? If you prefer to relax or straighten your hair, don't let anyone else's preconceived ideas about what ethnic women should or shouldn't do, or should or shouldn't look like, limit your style. Plus, you might not know that there's historic precedent: In ancient African custom, women routinely smoothed their hair with mud clay in order to weigh it down and straighten it. Today, if you decide you want to change or reshape your natural curl or wave pattern, here are your options.

RELAXERS

Before I go any further, I must stress to you how strongly I feel about going to a professional to relax your hair, versus doing it yourself. Doing it yourself can be tempting, especially if you're like me and have had your hair straightened, on and off, ever since you were a little girl. How hard can it be, you may think? But I've burnt my forehead and ears enough to know that it's best to let the professionals do it. I learned my lesson on a movie shoot, no less, when I tried to touch up my hair myself. Before I knew it, I had left the relaxer on too long and ended up burning out all the hair around my hairline (I had to resort to headbands for the rest of the film).

I think all of us know that the excessive use of relaxers can be hard on hair. The most typical misuse is not stopping with regrowth only. But despite risks like hair damage and breakage, relaxing one's hair using the chemical sodium hydroxide is still the most popular straightening procedure we use today. Quick, relatively easy (in a pro's hands, that is), it softens and changes the texture of the hair, allowing it to be transformed into dozens of different styles.

Part of the popularity of chemical relaxing stems from the fact that pressing one's hair offers only temporary effects that

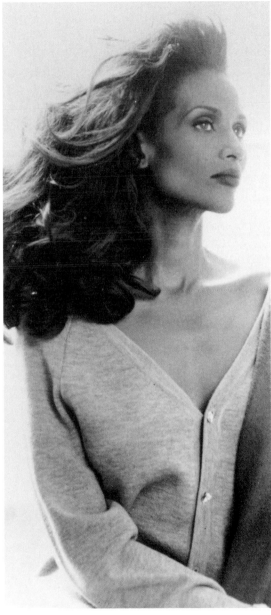

When my hair is relaxed, I just wash, condition and set it for soft, flowing waves like this.

TIP

Some caveats to keep in mind

Don't try to color and relax hair at the same time, particularly in an at-home situation. Even when this is done by the pros, it can be risky at best. Most experts recommend straightening the hair first, waiting at least two weeks, and then having the coloring done in a reputable salon that has experience with African-American hair. Since I've lightened my hair, I don't even risk chemical relaxing anymore and strongly advocate using a straightening iron (sometimes called a pressing iron or hot comb), followed by a curling comb for styling.

◆

If swimming is your favorite exercise, take care to protect your chemically relaxed hair from the chemicals in chlorinated pools, which can cause breakage and discoloration. Before swimming, comb a good conditioner through your hair, then tuck your hair under a bathing cap. After swimming, immediately shampoo to wash out chlorine; follow up with a leave-in conditioner. Tip: Comb wet hair very gently always and never pull it back into a chignon or pony tail. Wet hair shrinks as it dries, and you risk too much breakage that way.

◆

The stress on the hair from too-tight relaxer rollers can also cause you to lose hair around the margins of the scalp. This is a condition called traction alopecia—thank goodness, it's usually only temporary.

◆

Try to avoid combing through your hair while it's being straightened. The straightening process affects the hair's natural elasticity. When it's combed out, it may stretch out to over twice its length—and then break!

◆

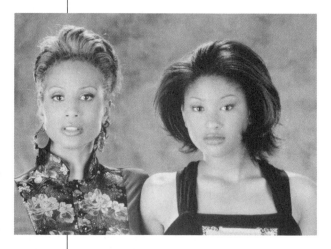

Two similar looks, but with two different treatments. Because lightened hair like mine shouldn't be relaxed, I used a straightening comb for this sleek do. Anansa, on the other hand, went the relaxing route: her hair is thoroughly conditioned, then brushed softly back.

One of the best—and most workable styles: hair that's blow-dryed, straightened at the edge with a straightnening comb, and softly framing the face. It's clean, easy, always sophisticated.

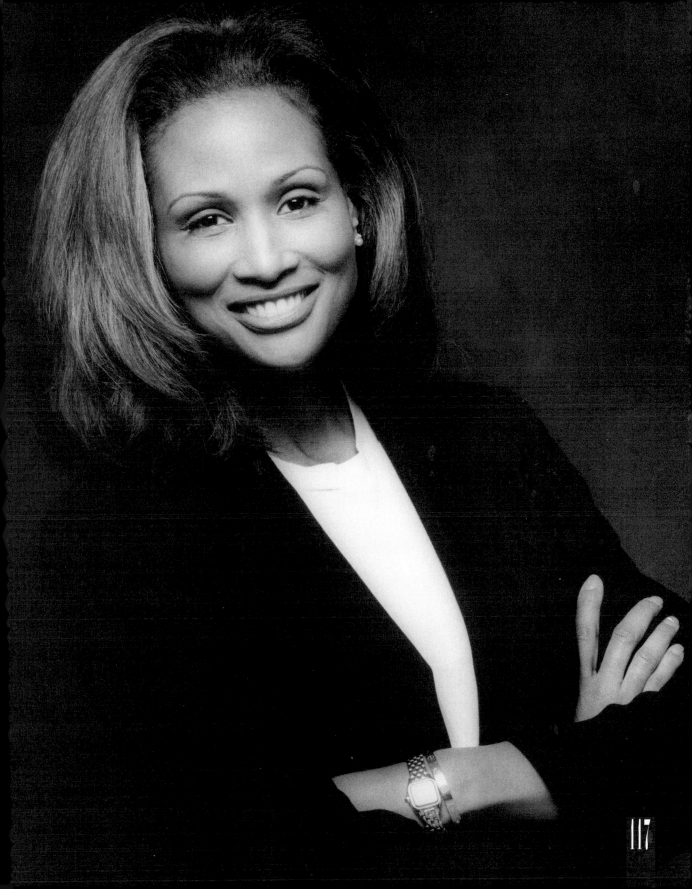

117

often don't last from shampoo to shampoo or when you perspire. Plus, pressing can be difficult to do by yourself, as is relaxing, unless you're very good with your hair. Once again, for best results with either process, it's always best to have a professional do it for you.

Even if you're having your hair relaxed in a salon, it's a good idea to know how the process works: First, clean, dry hair is saturated with the relaxing solution, then combed through and pulled straight. The relaxer is left on for a specified amount of time, according to the manufacturer's directions (usually around eight minutes) and depending on how strong your own curl is and how straight you want your hair to be. The longer the relaxing solution is left on, the longer the effects will last. After the relaxer is rinsed off and the hair shampooed, a neutralizer is added to stop the relaxing process and restore the pH balance to the hair. Finally, the neutralizer is rinsed out, and the hair is conditioned, gently towel-dried, and rolled in curlers.

Because the relaxing solution can be harsh, most hair experts recommend having a strand test before going through with the procedure. If your hair is very fine, for instance, a milder solution left on for a shorter amount of time might be in order; if your hair is strong, a stronger solution may be fine. Because there are so many variables, it's really a good idea to have your hair relaxed in a salon, and let the professionals judge. Be sure your stylist applies Vaseline or conditioner around the hairline to protect your skin from the relaxing solution. You can also ask your stylist about using a milder solution but leaving it on longer, and taking special efforts to keep it off the scalp.

Typically, relaxing lasts up to six months, depending on your hair texture and growth, and most experts agree that hair should be relaxed no more than every three months. Just keep in mind that it is best to go to a salon for any chemical process. After all, while relaxing makes hair more manageable and easier to control, one misstep can cause terrible hair damage as well.

PERMS

Perming African-American hair has become yet another "straightening" technique, one that's fast replacing others as a way to transform frizzy hair (that has not already been straightened or relaxed) into the kind of soft waves that allow for easier maintenance and more styling freedom. With a "curly perm," hair can be worn loose and casual by day, then slicked back and set in waves at night.

The perm process is essentially the same as relaxing except for the type of chemical used. **How it's done:** A solution (usually ammonium thioglycolate) is applied to clean, dry hair, which is then set on large rods. After a specific time according to manufacturer's directions (usually around twenty minutes, depending on the amount of natural curl in your hair), neutralizer is added to close the cuticle. The result: Tight natural curls become looser and softer.

Because of all the variables involved—and the risk of damage to the hair—a perm, like conventional relaxing, is definitely a salon procedure.

Every year salons come up with more techniques that can make your hair work for you. Texturizing, for example, loosens the natural curl only slightly, so the hair remains wavy (this process is very popular with men). It's a somewhat gentler procedure that allows for smooth blow-drying results. As one expert put it, "It lets us comb through our hair with a fine-tooth comb!"

PERMS AND COLOR FOR ASIAN, LATIN, NATIVE AMERICAN, AND INDIAN HAIR

In general, due to the tightness of the hair cuticle, as well as the hair's thickness and coarseness, perms (and coloring) have often been harder for Asian, Latin, Native American, and Indian women. However, new techniques, such as the availability of pre-softeners, are making them much easier.

Asian women in particular like to have their hair permed in order to vary its super-straight texture. But traditionally it's been thought that Asian hair won't "take" perming well and that extra-strong solutions for hard-to-curl hair were in order. In some cases, though, only the initial perm is hard and subsequent ones get much easier. A good idea is to use a pre-softener to "roughen up" the cuticle and make it easier to penetrate. How this works: Apply a perm solution or color to the hair, rinsing it out without styling; then a few weeks later, complete the process doing the actual perm (or color) a second time. The first application breaks down or roughens the cuticle enough so that the second application will set easier. Note: There are times when Asian hair will "take" a perm very quickly and a solution that's too strong or that's left on too long will burn and damage the hair. Since you don't know how your hair is going to react, it's always best to do a strand test first, and to perm in a carefully controlled salon setting only.

119

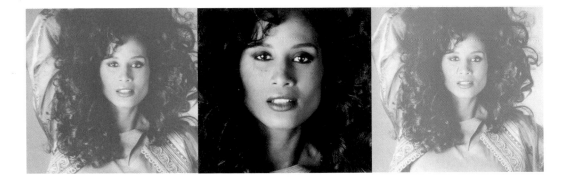

Your hair
can also
be an
expression
of your
sensuality—
when it's
wild and
tumbled
like this...

Tip: For a temporary curl in super-straight Asian hair for a special appointment or evening out), after letting your hair dry 60 percent, take half-inch segments of hair and twist them the entire length; then apply long, bendable foam-covered curlers. Let dry, remove curlers, and gently comb.

STRAIGHTENING TOOLS

Pressing is the oldest way to make excessively curly hair straight. Once considered old-fashioned and hard to do, it is having an enormous resurgence these days. Particularly if you color your hair, as I do, a straightening iron (also known as a hot comb) is actually a healthier option than chemical relaxing techniques; although it takes some practice to do it well, it is certainly worth a try. Besides, today, with electric straightening irons (as opposed to the old, on-the-stove variety, which were hard to use and control), the whole process is much easier. **Note:** Never hot comb chemically relaxed hair, even only at the roots.

How it's done: First be sure that your hair is dry and absolutely clean so that no soap, shampoo, or soil residue gets baked into your hair. Usually pomade is put on the hair from root to ends, then a hot pressing iron (also called a straightening iron) is applied to pull out (or "iron") the curl. Because the heat of the iron heats the pomade or hair oil

Tip:

When you style your hair with heat—whether with a pressing comb, curling iron, or blow dryer—the correct temperature for heat-styling appliances is 300°F to 350°. Hair begins to singe from 350°to 470°(at this temperature, white paper turns brown and may burst into flames). Needless to say, the hair's cuticle layers become burned, the ends split, and the hair's keratin is destroyed.

you use, take care not to let the hot oil trickle down the hair shaft; hot oil can burn the scalp, injure the hair follicle, and cause scar tissue and even hair loss. It's also important to keep the pomade or hair oil away from the skin around your hairline where it can cause a flare-up of acne, and to carefully control the heat of the iron so you don't burn or singe your hair. **Note:** If you're like me and don't care to have your hair "weighed down" with pomade, try pressing it without pomade, using an iron that's not quite so hot. After pressing, you can put curl back in, if you want to, with a curling iron. While pressing does indeed straighten hair and eliminate frizz, the results are only temporary, and it does "wash out" after shampooing (or when the weather is very humid).

COLORING YOUR HAIR

Like many women, I like to change my hair color from time to time. There's probably no easier way to make a dramatic difference in the way you look than a change in hair color. Even a subtle change—say a shade or two lighter or darker—can make a noticeable difference in your appearance. As your hair begins to gray and if you decide to color it, always go for a color a little lighter than your natural shade (it's softer and more flattering near the face), as opposed to one that's a shade or two darker, which can look harsh and artificial.

Today, on the whole, there is a much wider range of color options for any woman of color who wants to color her hair—wonderful burgundy tones, deep mahogany, rich, burnished browns, tawny reds. In most cases, your most flattering shade won't be too far afield from your natural color. A good rule of thumb: Top colorists always suggest going no more than four levels lighter. Steer clear of pitch-black shades, which are harsh and aging or you may end up looking like Morticia!

Before you decide on a hair color, consider carefully how it complements your skin tone. I find that warm red or auburn tints, for instance, can add warmth and brightness to olive or yellowish skin tones, while dark, warm browns or dark auburn shades can be vibrant and rich with dark-brown coloring. If your skin is on the lighter side—golden or bronze—think about a coppery shade or a sun-washed brown. Both can be extremely flattering and surprisingly "natural."

It's also important to consider your natural hair color as well. For example, if your hair is naturally very dark, it probably has a good deal of red pigment in it. This will only become more noticeable when your hair is lightened. To minimize red tones, choosing a color fairly close to your natural shade is your best bet.

Asian women often look best with cooler-toned tints in their hair, such as burgundy, plum, black cherry, or blue-reds. Latin women tend to look best with warmer tones like copper, bronze, or gold.

Probably the best way to determine your ideal hair color is to have a professional consultation and pick out some colors you like. Check them out at home by draping your head with a similarly hued scarf or even a piece of construction paper. **Note:** If your hair has been chemically relaxed, stay away from a very light hair color shade, and always wait at least four weeks between treatments for best results.

COLOR WITH CARE

I strongly advise visting a salon to have your hair colored rather than going the at-home route: Once again, it's just too easy to inadvertently damage your hair. The fact

An easy, always flattering way to control hair in a pinch—with a classic headband (that's the solution Anansa and I both turned to on a recent trip to Africa).

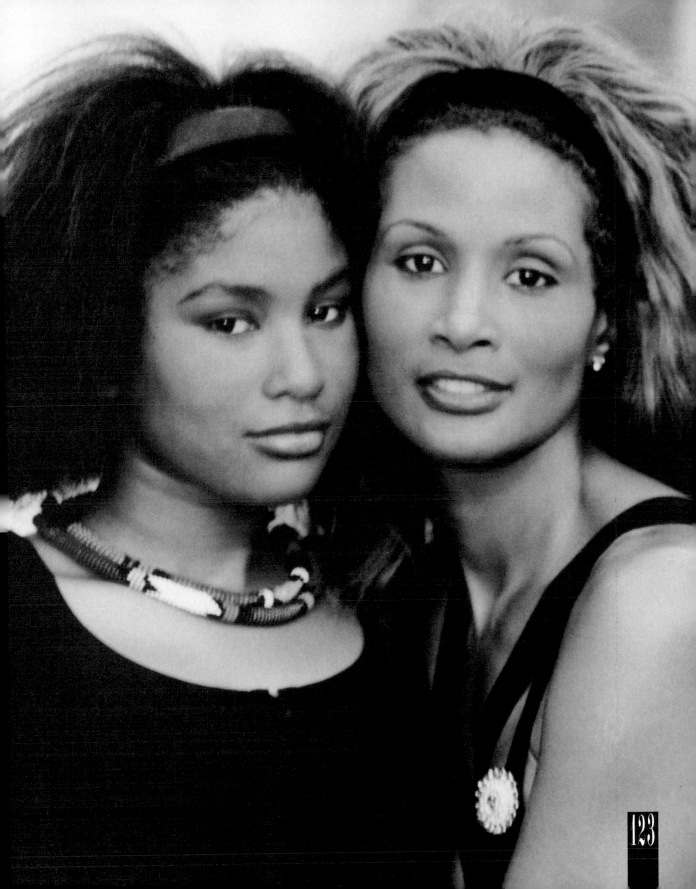

ALTERNATIVE COLORING TECHNIQUES FOR ETHNIC HAIR

Temporary color, meaning color treatments that don't penetrate the hair shaft, can give darker ethnic hair a boost of color on a short-term basis. These usually take the form of a rinse, and are either naturally or chemically derived (although without the peroxide or ammonia used in permanent tints).

Semi-permanent color (and now even demi-permanent color, which is a little stronger) gives a lovely translucent color to dark hair, which can look dull with a more opaque tint. Where a permanent dye strips the hair's natural color, then adds new color, these semi-permanent colors deposit color on top of your hair's natural shade, so they can really enhance or brighten your hair without overstripping.

Vegetable dyes give a subtle boost—and a lot of shine—but because they're naturally derived (not chemical), they stay only on the hair's surface and don't penetrate deep into ethnic hair. That means they're best for temporary color. Fruits, berries especially, make the best "vegetable" dyes, and dark hair can be beautifully enhanced by blackberry (which adds a burgundy shine), blueberry (a blue-black shine), or raspberry (a slightly red tint). Carrots and currants also give a nice red.

is that African-American hair loses color easily and timing can be very tricky. When you do go, be sure to choose a salon where the colorist is not only experienced in general, but familiar with African-American hair and the way it reacts to different types of color. Request products with a minimum of peroxide because anything too strong can easily cause your hair to break. **Note:** Henna, while certainly a natural coloring substance, is really not a good idea for African-American hair; it often leaves it dry and straw-like, especially when used with some other chemical treatment, like a perm.

Asian, Latin, Native American, and Indian hair, all traditionally hard to color, usually benefit from pre-softening to help the hair "hold" the color (see page 119). The color solution should be applied twice; the first application breaks down the cuticle, the second "sets" the color.

In addition, color solutions for these types of darker hair shouldn't be opaque—too covering—but translucent: Color washes or color rinses can bring up beautiful tonal qualities in ethnic hair, rather than cover them up. About peroxide: High levels of peroxide are definitely to be avoided, but some peroxide does assist the breakdown of hair, which allows color solutions to take hold. Color solutions with low levels of peroxide are best, and never use a solution that contains both ammonia and peroxide, which can result in a reddish tinge. Store-bought rinses, by the way, are often too opaque and won't match your hair tone exactly.

Most stylists these days prefer highlighting to all-over color: It's prettier, it's less boring, and, most important, it's less damaging to the hair since the whole head isn't colored. Because African-American hair absorbs rather than reflects light (which means it doesn't have much natural shine), highlights can also add brilliance and depth to hair that looks flat and dull. A beautiful sunny brown, for example, can add life to black hair and still have a natural look.

CAN YOU COLOR AND STRAIGHTEN?

Can you safely color and straighten? Yes, but only with care. First of all, it's important to wait several weeks—preferably a month—after straightening your hair before attempting color. That's because not only do relaxer chemicals cause stress to your hair, they may also lighten it slightly as well. In addition, if you color your hair too soon after straightening, your hair may "take," or absorb, the color too quickly and turn out too dark. **Tips:** Prior to adding color, deep condition your chemically

Note: What about doing these fruit dyes at home? Although it may sound like fun, it's really not such a good idea. You can grind up fresh raspberries or blackberries, and work them through your hair, but if your hair is dark, the results will probably be even more temporary than salon fruit rinses (which have added hair penetrators). If your hair is light, the fruit juice might stain unevenly. Best bet: Ask to try a fruit-based rinse at your favorite salon. Herbal tea rinses, on the other hand, are easy to do at home. While generally not strong enough to affect the color of ethnic hair, they can do wonders as conditioning rinses. Just brew up some chamomile tea and use it for a soothing final rinse. Nettle has healing qualities, and comfrey can be soothing to the scalp. And all give the hair wonderful shine.

My mother's beauty routines are well-thought out...and always changing (different looks work at different moments in your life). These days, she prefers to color the gray in her relaxed hair, then give it a quick set and a blow dry.

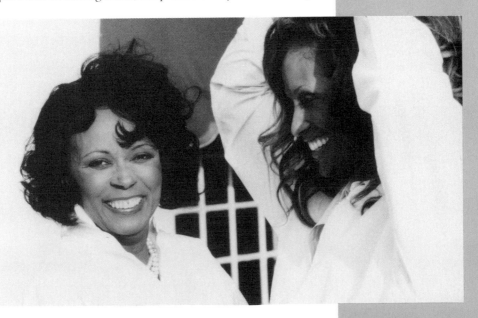

straightened hair twice a week for several weeks. Never straighten your hair immediately after coloring either, as the straightener may strip the color from your hair, leaving it faded.

Another color solution that works for chemically treated hair is to try a no-ammonia, no-peroxide color such as Sebastian's Cellophanes Plus. This type of hair color, which is gentler on the hair, moisturizes as well as adds shine, and can actually help leave your hair in better condition than when you started.

Asian women, whose hair is traditionally considered hard to color because of its tight cuticle, should also always go to a pro if they want to try a little color to vary their look. Subtle burgundy highlights, for example, can add a beautiful "light" to a natural, deep sable-brown color. There are also new pre-coloring products—called "softeners"—like Cellophanes Plus SX (Special Effects), which have been developed especially for hard-to-penetrate Asian and Latin hair. These products "roughen up" the cuticle to help it absorb more color.

COVERING GRAY

There are two ways to deal with gray hair: Either wear it with pride—or color it. It's as simple as that. When I was a little girl I used to picture myself as an older lady with two long, silver-white braids down my back. Well, I still may go for those long braids, but they're not going to be silver white anymore! The fact is that in this country we tend to instantly associate gray hair with age.

If you have gray in your hair that you prefer to cover, many experts suggest blending the gray in with your natural color by using a temporary rinse or semi-permanent hair color. If you choose a shade one or two tones lighter than your natural color, your own color won't be affected, but the gray will appear as very attractive highlights.

Black women tend to gray later in life than Caucasians. If you decide to leave your hair gray, wear that color with pride and distinction. Do keep in mind, however, that if you straighten your hair, excessive heat from straightening combs can yellow the color, which is something you don't want.

Asian women, who generally go gray quite slowly, should avoid using jet-black rinses or tint to cover their gray; they tend to make the hair color too flat and dull. If your hair is black, go for the darkest brown (but not black) that you can find. If your hair is medium brown, try to find a matching tone, but without too much red in it.

There are two ways to deal with gray hair: either wear it with pride— or color it. It's as simple as that.

As a general rule for gray hair for all ethnic types, keep in mind that your gray hairs may often be a totally different texture from hair with color; they're usually quite wirey and can be unruly. This means that as you gray, it's probably a good idea to consider moisture-based products, such as a moisturizing shampoo, and firmer-hold gels and styling products.

STYLE AND CUT

No question, African-American hair is very trend-oriented. There are just a tremendous number of beautiful and creative ways to wear our hair. If you have the confidence to do so, by all means experiment with all the new looks that come in, with braids as elaborate as the headdress of a high priestess, with hair-lengthening extensions and upswept curls. Anansa, like most teenagers, adores experimenting with her hair. She'll part it down the middle, put on a hairpiece or a switch, try bangs, a Dutchboy, fine Shirley

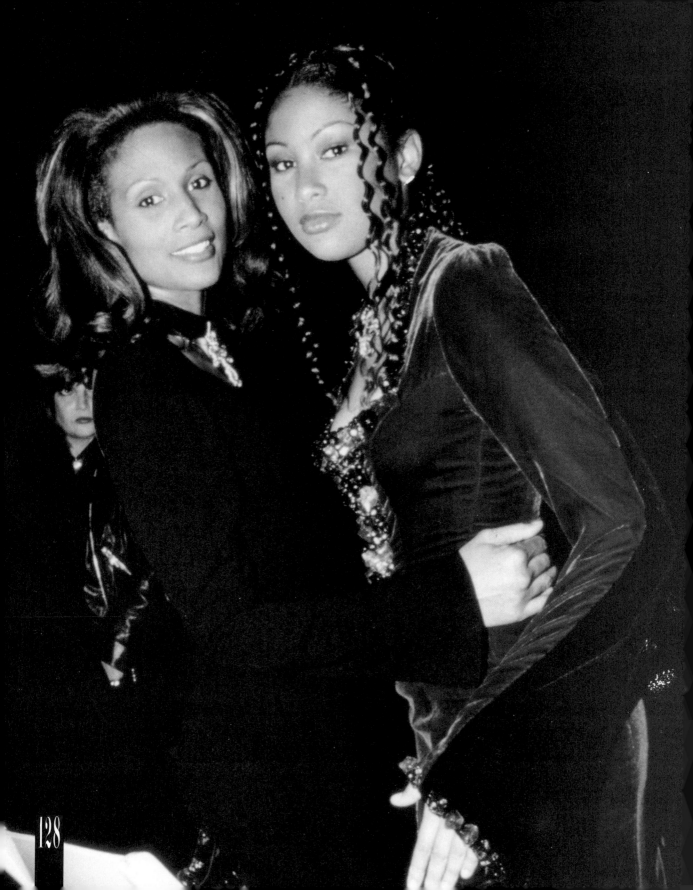

Temple curls—you name it. And why not? That's the beauty of our beautiful hair.

When people ask me about what kinds of styles I think are appropriate for African-American hair and what kinds aren't, I generally have one answer: I don't believe you should limit your imagination in regards to style. Try the unexpected—have fun with your hair! With the blossoming of the awareness of African roots in the past decade, for instance, has come the rediscovery and enjoyment of all sorts of African-inspired hairstyles, especially tiny braids arranged in intricate designs. Particularly these days, when contemporary high style and African style creatively mix—even in the boardroom—forming various original looks, the results can be extraordinary.

Like most of us, I love to try out different looks, especially for evening. But there's another issue to keep in mind here and that's length. As women get older, I often find they look better in shorter hairstyles, not because long hair is suitable only for young women—it's not—but because shorter hair can be softer-looking. A slightly longer than chin-length cut often works well on older women because it "lifts" the features and clears the neck and chin line. Yet it's still long enough to comb back into a chignon for a sophisticated evening look.

I don't believe you should limit your imagination in regards to style. Try the unexpected...have fun with your hair.

Your choice of a style will also have to take into account how much time you're willing to devote to your hair. Most women in the working world, for example, find that a simple blunt cut has the kind of low maintenance they're looking for, as opposed to a layered cut that requires blow drying and setting. Whatever you choose, use your common sense and best judgment as to what's appropriate for your work situation. **Note:** Keep in mind that certain hairstyles can actually harm the hair, leading to scalp damage, infection, and even permanent hair loss. Braids, for example, should never be worn so

Anansa and me—at her first benefit fashion show. My hair is soft and waved; she's trying out a flirty pin-on hairpiece of corkschrew curls.

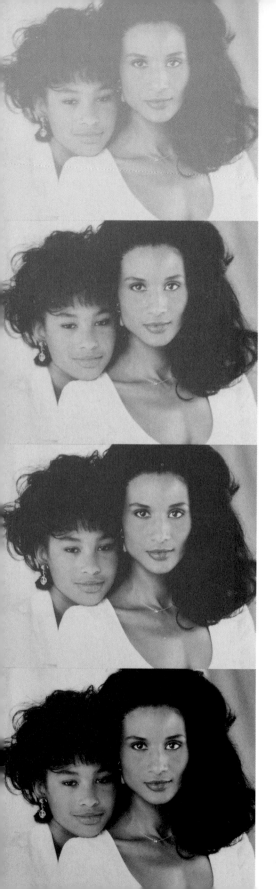

tightly that they cause stress and pull on the scalp. The tension caused by the very tight braids often worn by little girls can pull the hair so much that the hair follicle becomes open to bacterial infection.

If you have a beautiful head shape and a long neck, a natural, sculptured style can be a clean and elegant look—such cuts can be worn blown straight, or natural, or parted in any number of ways (and should be trimmed about every two weeks to keep their shape). A touch of pomade is also a good idea to help the hair keep its shape and to enhance the shine, plus a moisturizer and leave-in conditioner to help keep the hair as healthy as possible.

WHAT YOU NEED TO KNOW ABOUT BRAIDING, HAIR WEAVING, HAIR EXTENSIONS, BONDING, AND HAIR BUYING

African-inspired braids—tightly woven into intricate patterns, in exquisite spiraled cornrows and unique designs—create one of the most glamorous looks I've tried over the years, and one that takes full advantage of the texture and properties of our hair. Going far beyond the ubiquitous cornrow styles of the 1970's, today's styles are complex, artistic, and time-consuming. Depending on the style and the part of the country you live in, braiding by a specialist can take

Simple, elegant hairstyles can take you from work to an evening out.

How do you wear your hair when you're riding on an elephant? Like a lioness, of course!

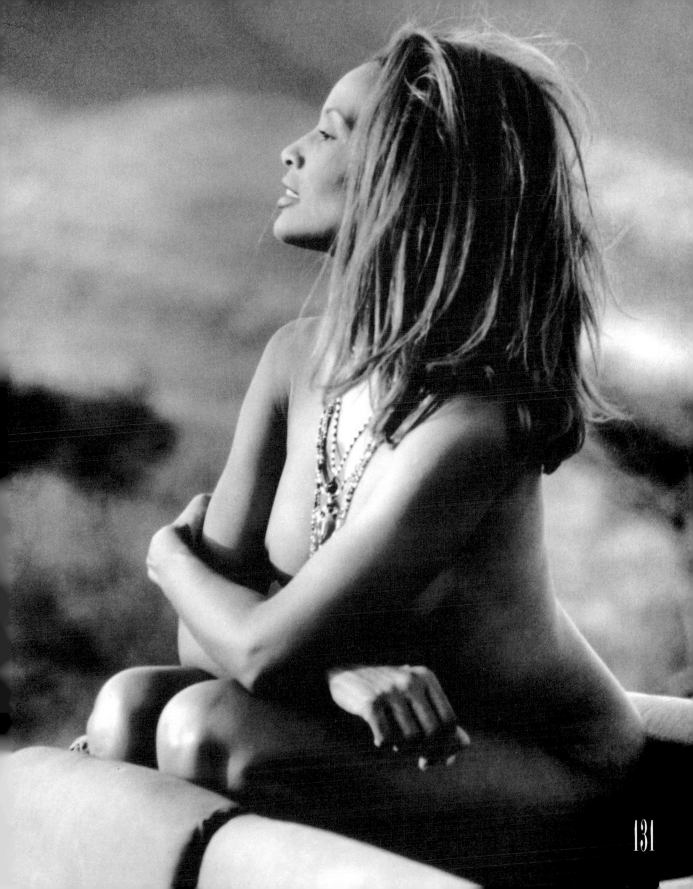

TIP

Any suggestions about buying and caring for a wig?

Wigs are great timesavers for busy women. When I was younger, I was more into working with just my own hair, which is fine. These days, though, I love to experiment with different styles, shapes, and colors, and since this is easiest to do without lopping off my own hair, I do it with wigs. I have short, pixie-like wigs, curly wigs, bob-length wigs, wigs in natural colors, and even a few in platinum blonde. Anansa, like most young women, likes her own hair, but from time to time, she is fascinated with my wigs and even wore one of the long, curly ones for a modeling test!

◆

For the most natural-looking results, I recommend buying a wig at a beauty salon or from a wig specialist, then having it cut and styled by your hairstylist to complement your own features and head shape, and to achieve the most natural look around the hairline. Also before you buy be sure to check out how it looks from the front, back, and sides, and then get an overview in a full-length mirror.

◆

Synthetic wigs are less costly and easier to maintain than those made from human hair. For the most comfort (and coolness), look for ones with an inner cap that breathes, with open netting or crisscrossed strands or ribbon. Note: To care for a synthetic wig, brush with a wire brush before washing. Then cold-water wash it in the sink. Rinse well in cold water and pat dry, then shake out to style. Don't use a hair dryer, comb, or brush when wet.

◆

anywhere from six to thirty hours, and cost from $250 to $750. (Rope-like dreadlocks, by the way, while not actually braids, are part of the braid family. The hair is washed, dried, and twisted, but otherwise left in its natural state.)

Hair extensions and hair weaving, phenomena of the last decade, have also moved into the mainstream and become more sophisticated than ever. These provide a longer, fuller, healthier-looking hairstyle, with only minimal stress and maintenance. I love to have extensions added to my hair, even when my own hair is a fairly good length, just to enhance that fabulous, wild lioness look. I adore the idea of walking around with an incredible mane of hair—it couldn't possibly be real, but it doesn't matter because it looks absolutely gorgeous! Of course a look like this doesn't come easily—or quickly: For me, it involved a twelve-hour sitting (during which time I read every magazine in the place). My hair ended up reaching all the way down to the small of my back—not uncomfortable, by any means, but definitely a feeling I had to get used to.

Especially if you're active, extensions or weaving can be convenient after a workout or a swim (particularly in the summer when you don't want to fuss with your hair).

While the words "extensions" and "weaving" are sometimes used interchangeably, there is actually a difference in technique. With extensions (braids), your hair is braided at the scalp, then individual extensions (commercial hair, either human or synthetic) are braided or sewn into the natural hair. A wool fiber from west Africa is used to make some styles fuller and longer-lasting.

Weaving, on the other hand, begins by cornrowing or twisting (interlocking) sections of hair at the scalp as a base to which wefted hair (extensions that are sewn onto a weft) is sewn. Although braids produce less stress, wefted hair does provide more height and drama (often experts will use both techniques on one head of hair). I personally find weaving to be a *little* more uncomfortable, although I put up with it because of the truly fabulous fullness it can achieve (it's something I'll do, for instance,

Asian Hair: Because Asian hair is so straight, every cut shows, unlike with curly or wavy hair, where the cut mark is absorbed into the wave. That's why layered cuts seldom work on Asian or straight hair, and why one-length blunt cuts are so elegant and attractive. Some stylists also suggest that Asian women steer clear of extremely short hair because the straightness of the hair makes it tend to spring up when cut too short. What does works: In any cut, leave it a little bit longer than other hair types because it needs the extra weight in order to fall neatly into place. For example, with a short cut or a shag, the nape can be cut short or tapered, but the top should be left a little longer so that it falls correctly.

For longer cuts, angling works well. Hair can be cut at an angle, with the back a little longer, then curving upward toward the front. A "texturizing sheer" can also be used. This notches the hair slightly (rather than the fine line that a scissors gives) and helps hair fall evenly in a straight line.

For Wavy/Curly Hair (Latin): When cutting this type of hair, it's best not to use a lot of tension when holding the hair before cutting—curly hair will spring back after being held,

for a really special occasion, like the premiere of a big movie). In a way, too, it's actually better for your hair since your own hair is cornrowed up and doesn't undergo any wear and tear. Plus it gets a chance to grow.

Hair bonding is another way to achieve the look of longer hair, but it's one that many stylists and hair experts suggest avoiding. I agree. This sort of hair extension method can be damaging to African-American hair since it utilizes glue or melted synthetic hair to "bond" with the natural hair, causing damage.

Most people find extensions can look natural and wear well. Some women, Latin as well as African-American, do like to buy their own hair for extensions (or for falls and wiglets). Such hair is usually sold by the ounce by commercial suppliers who purchase it in bulk. At the supplier, strands of hair are pulled out of skeins and custom-blended to match your own. If you feel you're knowledgeable enough about matching the color and texture of your hair, by all means do so; otherwise leave the purchase to your stylist, who probably can find the best match for your hair. Synthetic hair is often used more than human because it holds curls and waves better (and it's especially good for a very tight braid).

The results of any of these processes last between three and five months, ideal if you're looking for a low-maintenance style. Extensions are also terrific for those who want the look of long, luxurious hair while allowing their own hair to grow leaving it much shorter than intended. Ask your stylist for a "low-tension" cut to ensure the length you want. Also, to really play up curly hair, you can "volumize" it—tilt the head to one side, comb the hair through the fingers and hold it up, then spray with hair spray at the roots. Hold for a minute to dry, then release.

out. **Tip:** Most stylists recommend that you let no more than three or four months go by between weavings or your hair will matte and you won't be able to comb it out.

After the investment of time and money, the key to these looks is maintenance. Most styles that require extensions or weaving can be washed (not those with wool extensions, though), but the emphasis is on care and cleanliness of the scalp, not the hair. **How to:** Shampoo as usual with a moisturizing shampoo (a clear gel usually works best; avoid heavy creams that can get embedded in the scalp and cause flaking). If conditioning is needed, thin a little gel with hairdressing cream and dab it directly on the scalp. As your hair grows out, extensions are either tightened or removed by simply cutting the hair where your natural braid ends, then shampooing thoroughly but gently with a cream-based product. **Tip:** Because your own hair is mixed in with the extension, it's important to be gentle when you comb. Remember, it's your own hair that you'll be breaking if you don't take the time to condition and comb carefully. As for shampooing braids, don't rub the hair vigorously, but do rinse it thoroughly. It's amazing what water will do.

♦

Celebrating the New Beauty—
and Beauties—of Color

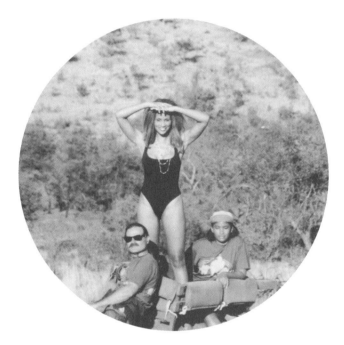

The photos in this section tell a story of sorts—and happily it's a success story—of just how many different ways there are for women of color to look these days and just how far we've come. The fact is, when I was growing up in the 1970's, African-American women were only starting to make their presence known in the modeling world. And somehow, the unspoken rules of the game "decreed" that there could be only one so-called superstar model of color at a time (and usually no more than one ethnic model on a shoot). In other words, if we were black...or Asian...or Latin...we seldom got to work with our peers.

On the beach, and completely natural. Hair just washed and dried. Not much makeup either: a dab of mascara, slicked on sun protection (always).

137

When hair goes lighter, adjust your makeup as well. Here pale, sun-blushed colors, all in the same tone, create an appealing soft look.

A touch of color adds definition, shape, to rich, natural crinkles and waves.

139

All-out nighttime allure means the power of red—a strong mouth, stained a rich crimson, eyes rimmed in sooty grays, blacks...

Another knockout choice—the warm lights and subtle shine of bronze... a touch of gold shimmer dabbed on lips.

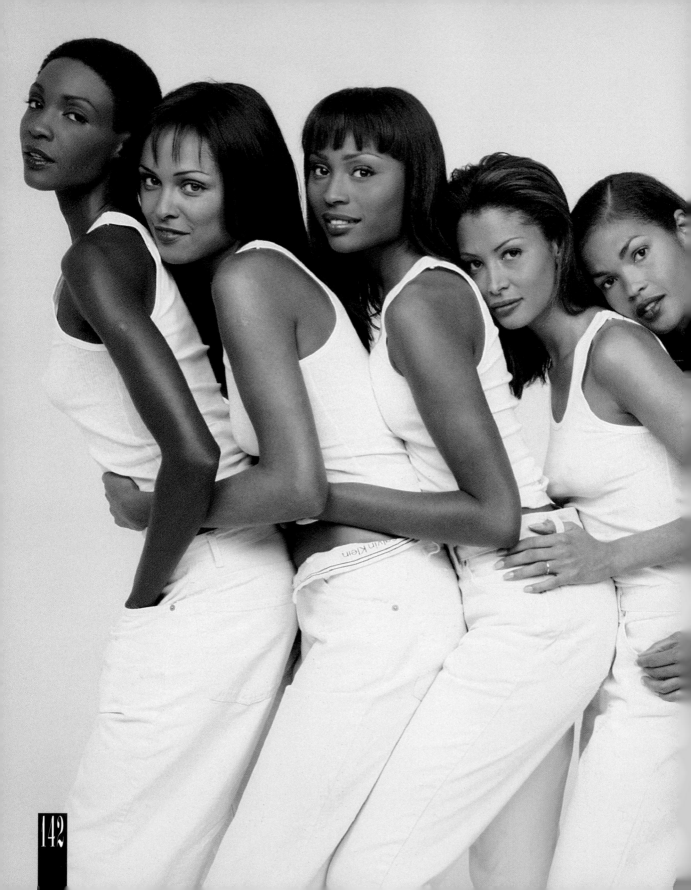

143

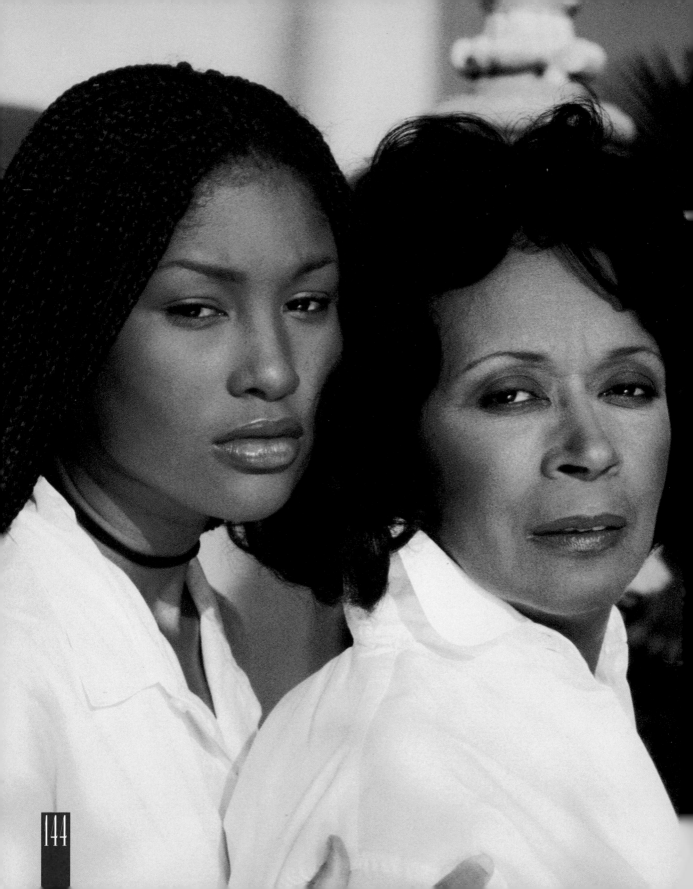

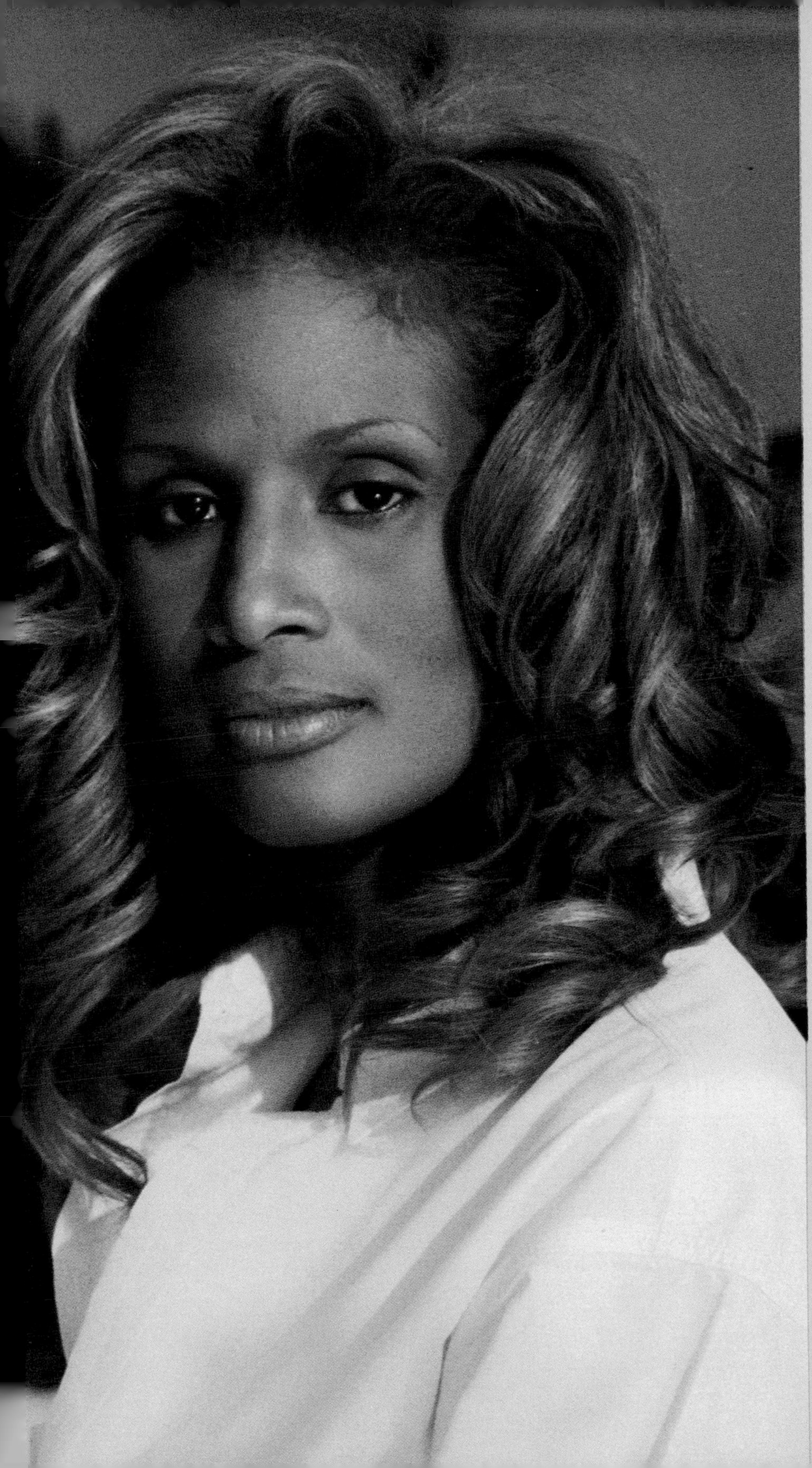

The look of three
generations—
three proud
women, three
different ages.
Each period in
your life will
have its own
beauty, vitality,
and allure.

Different moods call for different looks, makeup. Here's Anansa— wild curls, sultry makeup, a Carmen Miranda fantasy...

...or romantic,
demure—brows
arched, cuffs
awash in
Edwardian lace.

147

My own personal favorite look for evening—makeup that's dramatic yet understated, makeup layered on a golden base.

148

How different things are today when women of color are heralded as the most visible and powerful women in the fashion business, from the runways of Paris to the covers of the most prestigious magazines. Our look has redefined what's attractive and what's modern for women of every color, at any age.

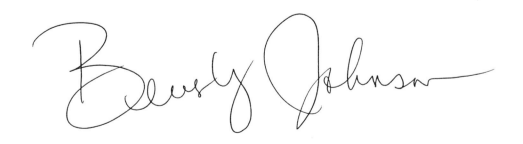

Beverly Johnson

FITNESS

for

Body

and

Soul

PART

II

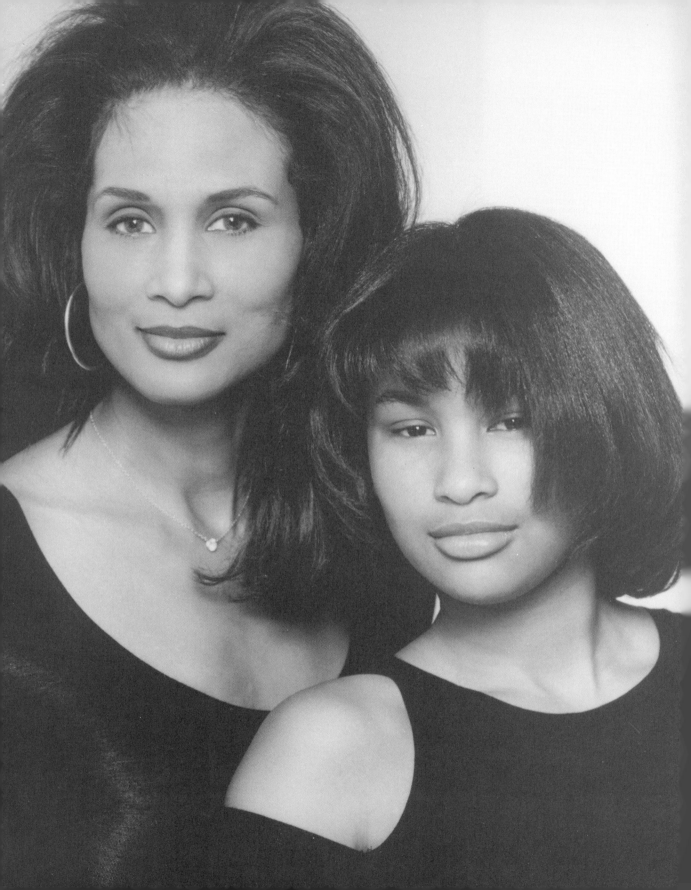

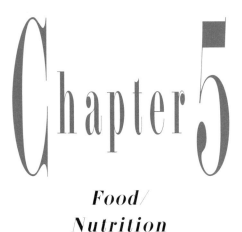

Chapter 5

Food/ Nutrition

Breaking the Diet Trap Once and for All

There was a time when a certain number on the scale was enough to demolish all my hard-won feelings of self-worth. I'm not going to tell you that number, but I will tell you that it's a quality about myself of which I'm not particularly proud. Still, remember this: Anyone who thinks that society pressures women in general to live up to an unrealistic ideal of perfect thinness can only imagine what models have to do to maintain that image. In this profession, one is constantly scrutinized and criticized for even the tiniest "flaws" (if you're at all sensitive, this is no place to be!). And the fact is that clothes do hang best on a hanger, so models have to struggle to look like one—broad shoulders, slim everywhere else—and that's no easy task.

Of course, now I know that I took extreme measures to control my weight, to the degree that I wound up anorexic and then bulimic—which are both life-threatening diseases (see page 181 for more on eating disorders). For me, it even got to the point that one day when I was visiting my mother back in Buffalo, she dragged me out of the shower and stood me in front of a three-way mirror. "What are you doing to yourself?" she pleaded. In fact, I looked like a Biafran. My ribs were sticking out. My arms looked like sticks. I started to cry.

Perhaps I should be embarrassed to admit it, but even that didn't bring me completely to my senses. Not yet. Even after seeing a nutritionist, it took years for me to work my way back to normal eating habits. But I did start this quest—learning about nutrition, vitamin supplements, and healthy eating. But somehow, it backfired: My whole system went out of whack and an uncontrollable anxiety come over me whenever I thought about food.

I became obsessed. I would sit down and eat doughnuts and whole pies. And because I knew I couldn't keep eating like this and work, I lapsed into bulimia, gorging myself one moment, purging the next. I was already a famous model, so being overweight wasn't handicapping me that much. (As many other well-known models at the top of their profession have done, I reached a point where I arrogantly insisted that clothes be slit down the back to fit me.) Besides, I thought, in a pinch I certainly knew how to take care of any temporary excess weight by purging before a big job. But what I wasn't facing was why I was doing this to myself and, despite the image of success I was presenting to the world, how unhappy and out of control I had become.

Whether it's getting a handle on your weight or your life, it all involves getting back to that strong spiritual and psychological center.

My moment of truth came one day as I was sitting in front of the TV at a friend's house, working my way through a box of doughnuts—and I mean big doughnuts. I began to panic. There is an enormous amount of pressure you're under when your job depends on your weight.

My friend, though, heard me in the bathroom, and the next thing I knew she insisted on taking me to my first meeting of a group called Overeaters' Anonymous. I listened—and shared my story with other people—and knew I was in the right place. Subsequently I also learned that as a result of my previous history of crash dieting, I had developed a thyroid problem that had contributed to the weight gain I had experienced.

As a result of the O.A. twelve-step program, although I know I will always

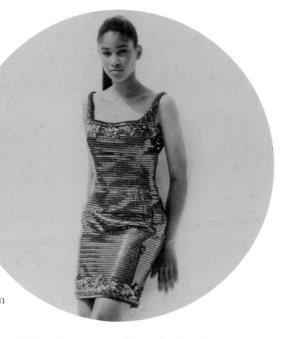

have an eating disorder, now I also know how to live and deal with it. And through education (educating myself not only nutritionally, but also emotionally and spiritually) I've reached a point where I can regard food differently. Sure, I may splurge on a couple of cookies now and then (even polish off a whole bag once in a while), but it's no longer the result of that ravenous, deprived feeling from which I once suffered.

There are so many reasons why some of us habitually overeat or binge during crises. Most have less to do with food than with emotional disturbances that interrupt our sense of well-being. That's why the key to establishing a successful and healthy eating pattern, once and for all, is understanding not only which foods to choose from (which I'll be talking about in the pages ahead), but also the psychological forces that trigger overeating in the first place.

Some of us turn to food as a sedative for our feelings, especially when it comes to sweets like candy and ice cream, or salty foods like pretzels and potato chips. Some of us turn to food to alleviate stress, or out of boredom or futility. There are so many reasons—lack of family support, sexual frustration (psycholgists often equate food and sex!), financial pressures, trouble at school, unfulfilling jobs or no jobs at all—that send us to the refrigerator for comfort.

But while eating should be pleasurable, satisfying the palate and sating the healthy appetite, it shouldn't be a source of emotional solace. There are better ways—and I'll

This photo of Anansa shows what a healthy body really looks like: toned, fit...and curvy.

155

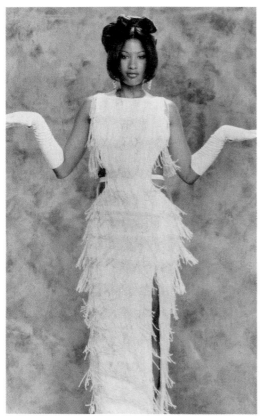

What you see is what you get—it's all about attitude and style. So whatever shape you're in, you can always walk tall—and proud.

talk about them—to relax or to feel good about yourself that don't involve reaching for a candy bar when you're unhappy or stressed out, or wolfing down a piece of chocolate cake to smooth over a bad mood or disappointment. As someone who has tried everything, from macrobiotic health foods to ultra-scientific eating regimens, I strongly believe that this is the key: Whether it's getting a handle on your weight or your life, it all involves getting back to that strong spiritual and psychological center.

THE CULTURAL FACTOR: ETHNIC WOMEN AND DIET

One of the special problems that women of color face in controlling our weight is that until recently we have had a distinctly cultural attitude about our bodies and dieting. In some ways, it's actually a positive thing. According to many studies, African-American (and Latin) women are generally proud of their bodies and satisfied with their appearance at higher weights than Caucasian women. While white women are considered "overweight," black women are "voluptuous." What this means is that we tend to "walk proud" even with that extra five, ten, or even twenty pounds. Indeed, according to *The Black Health Library Guide to Heart Disease,* "being overweight has been culturally accepted among many blacks—at least until recently—and even preferred by some. Who has not heard the age-old adage, "Nobody likes a bone but a dog"?

But attitudes are changing, as we become more and more aware of how important losing weight—and keeping it off—can be, not only for the sake of appearance, but to maintain our health. While certainly not everyone needs to be or should be fashion-model-thin (and the acceptance of healthy, feminine curves is, as I said, a strong and positive thing), the fact is that if you are very overweight, it's just no longer acceptable to say that you've come to terms with it and that's how you want to live the rest of your life, especially if your weight has reached the point where your health is affected by obesity-related ailments such as heart disease or hypertension. Pile on too many excess pounds on top of other risk factors, such as family history of high blood pressure or heart disease, add to that a sedentary lifestyle— and you've got a truly dangerous health threat that you should and must take seriously.

> ### What I advocate is reaching a mental place, a peace of mind where you are in control, and comfortable with the foods that you choose to eat. No guilt.

Once again, I'm not talking about trying to alter your body to suit someone else's idea of beauty. It's truly unfortunate that such eating disorders as anorexia and bulimia, which traditionally weren't ethnic problems, are now becoming more prevalent among young women of color who have grown up in assimilated environments. But I do believe that often we African-American women turn to food to anesthetize ourselves from our feelings—from the anxieties, stresses, and strife of life that we experience as women of color. The easy accessibility of greasy, high-fat, high-salt, and relatively inexpensive fast foods in many of our neighborhoods doesn't help, either. What I am talking about is

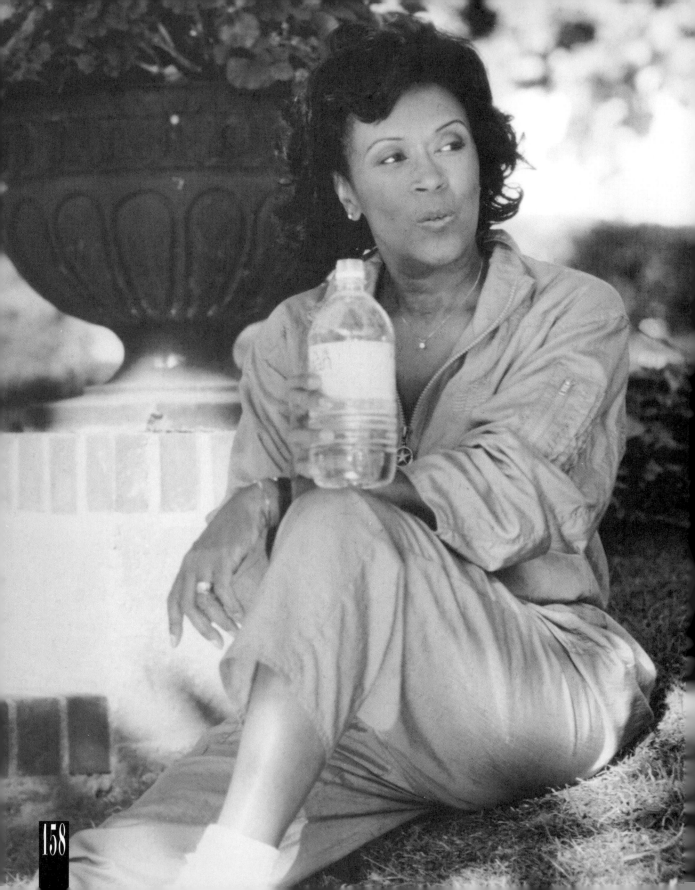

taking charge of your own health, your own body—and that includes your weight.

According to Jennifer Stack, R.D.N., who counsels women of color with dangerously high levels of blood sugar, cholesterol, and blood pressure, traditionally African-Americans have been reared on high-fat, high-salt diets—fried chicken, collard greens swimming in pork fat, lots of salt. Also in most societies it's the women who shop for and prepare almost all meals, who spend a good deal of time in the kitchen, and who naturally derive a good deal of self-esteem by presenting a bounteous and deliciously cooked spread of these traditional foods to our families and to guests in our homes.

But our children and husbands and boyfriends enjoy this kind of food, you may say. I know that when you see yourself as "mother," "cook," and "provider," it's hard to accept "depriving" your family. But by perpetuating what we now know are unhealthy eating habits, you could also be depriving your family of good health.

African-American women are not the only ones at risk for developing obesity-related diseases. While Latin diets are based on many healthful ingredients, such as rice, beans, and plantains, their benefits are canceled out by preparing them in fattening, unhealthy ways. Indians—even vegetarians—tend to use a lot of fat in food preparation as well. And Asians, who are traditionally brought up on low-fat, low-protein, high-carbohydrate diets, are beginning to develop the same problems, as they adopt Westernized eating habits. As a double whammy, Asians tend to acquire lactose intolerance (the inability to digest milk products) since milk products were not included in their traditional diets.

So what can you do? Actually a lot—and there's no better time to start than now. Modifying the meals you prepare for yourself and your family so that they are low in fat and high in complex carbohydrates (lots of fresh fruits, vegetables, and whole grains); incorporating some of the ideas and healthful changes I am going to be discussing; stocking up on healthy, natural treats instead of calorie-laden, high-fat snack foods—all can have a definite positive effect.

It's worth repeating...just how important water is to good looks and good health.

NEW NUTRITION FRONTIERS

What is the best way to lose weight and keep it off? I wish I had the easy answer—the magic secret, the ultimate foolproof diet that we're all looking for. But while there's always the temptation to go on that crash diet that promises quick weight loss in a short time, the fact is that we also know, in our heads, if not our hearts, that the results are only going to be temporary. Worse still, years of this sort of yo-yo dieting and "weight cycling" actually can slow your metabolism, making it harder than ever to lose weight.

With that in mind, the first and the most important thing that I want you to realize is that dieting—starving yourself and depriving yourself of food—is a thing of the past. Diets don't work. They never really have. Over the last decade, this has been conclusively proven again and again. I'm sure you know the routine: You lose the weight, you feel good. You gain it back again, you feel terrible. And, believe me, because I've done it myself, that is simply no way to live. So, let me repeat once again: *There just isn't anything positive to be achieved by dieting.*

Control

I want to say something here about "control," which is not a word you'll find me using when it comes to food and weight. The fact is that the idea of control—controlling your weight, controlling your diet—has a sense of rigidity to it, a harsh tyranny of discipline that I don't feel is compatible with how we really live our lives. The ritual of eating—breaking bread with our family and friends—should be a pleasure, not a chore, and should be approached with a sense of flexibility and flow.

What I advocate instead is reaching a mental place, a peace of mind where you are in control, and comfortable with the foods that *you* choose to eat—a mental state where you feel no guilt. If you can establish this, I believe you will actually enjoy eating in a way that you never have before. This is what I call becoming "centered" as far as the age-old obsession with weight and food are concerned. Have I reached this point myself? For the most part, yes—after a long struggle. And while in the back of my mind I probably will always feel I'm not at my ideal weight (part of this "disease" is that you never quite feel you're there), I have learned to trust the judgment of the people I love.

BEVERLY JOHNSON

So how can you get from where you are to this point? What are the steps, the strategies, the formulas to follow? Here I think I *can* help you get on the right track. Having been through a bout with eating disorders (and, let me emphasize, you're never cured; you only learn coping techniques), I've learned lots of different tactics that have helped me to reach my own personal goals. One of the most important, by the way, is not to chastise myself or Anansa when either of us occasionally strays from our good intentions. It happens. It certainly doesn't make me a "bad" or "unworthy" person or any such nonsense like that. I just accept that I'm only human—and fallible—and I go right back to a more positive way of eating.

A HEALTHY LIFETIME EATING PLAN

Without question, the best way to slim down is not to diet but to establish an eating plan you can stick with for the long run. If this sounds daunting and you're tempted to crash diet again, remember that after all the pain and effort of crash dieting, if you lose over two pounds a week the weight is only going to come back again.

Instead, think about a good, basic eating plan designed around satisfying portions of healthy, low-fat, high-fiber, high-bulk foods that make you feel full and not deprived. Foods in this category are typically fruits and vegetables, and whole-grain breads and cereals, which are high in complex carbohydrates to give you energy throughout the day. They also provide the

HERE ARE MY FOUR BASIC PRINCIPLES WHEN IT COMES TO HEALTHIER EATING AND BETTER NUTRITION:

- *Never let yourself get hungry. Eat low-fat snacks before sitting down to a meal (good choices: bagels, fresh fruit, low-fat cereal).*
- *Do not skip or skimp on meals. It's skipping meals—usually because you want to drop a few pounds or because you feel you overindulged at a previous meal—that can start you on the disastrous yo-yo diet syndrome you're trying to avoid.*
- *Increase your exercise. It's hard for me, too, but you've got to do it. Make it automatic, a given, like brushing your teeth every morning or washing your face.*
- *Think before you eat. What you eat is your choice.*

161

necessary calcium, iron, and fiber you need.

A good eating plan also has to be realistic, to take into account all the temptations and changes that real life has to offer (that's why I also build in some splurges and snacks along the way). After all, how many of you teenagers out there, even though you know better, still skip breakfast, skimp on lunch, and catch a fast-food dinner on the run? And in between fill in the gaps with snacks and soft drinks that have little, if any, nutritional value? It's exactly that kind of eating pattern, however, that leads to teenage weight problems, skin problems, and lack of energy overall.

Here is how I might approach a typical day of healthy eating:

Step 1: I like to have a fairly substantial breakfast. Typically, I might have two pieces of unbuttered whole-wheat toast, a serving of corn meal grits (with a pat of margarine

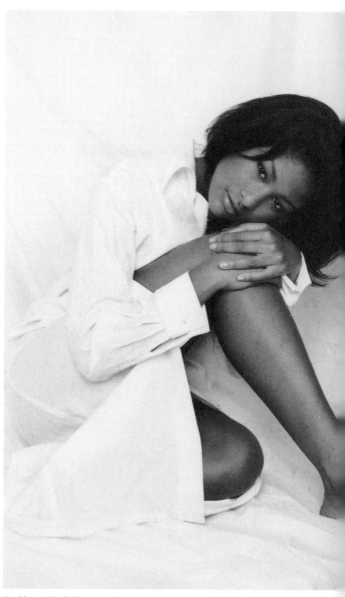

Healthy eating habits start in your teens (and a realistic approach includes a splurge now and then, too).

TIP

A healthy, real-life eating plan

For those of you who want a more structured eating plan, I consulted a nutritionist and put together this basic menu guide.

◆

Breakfast (approximately 260 calories)
1 cup 1% milk
1 cup whole-grain cereal

◆

Lunch (approximately 370 calories)
1 cup cooked whole-wheat pasta spirals
1 cup chopped green peppers, celery, carrots
2 tbs. low-calorie Italian dressing
3 oz. roasted or broiled white chicken meat
(added to pasta and vegetables)

◆

Dinner (approximately 380 calories)
1 cup barley or rice pilaf (without oil)
1 cup cooked collard greens or kale
1 tsp. olive oil for sautéing greens with garlic
2 oz. London broil or eye of round steak

◆

In addition, allow yourself three snacks each day. This might be two servings of fresh fruit and one serving of a calcium-rich food, such as 1 ounce of skim-milk cheese or 4 ounces of non-fat frozen yogurt. And every week splurge a little on a 200–300 calorie treat like a small order of French fries, a small fast-food hamburger, a small bag of potato chips, or a scoop of ice cream.

◆

I think you'll find this eating plan feasible, workable, and, most important, satisfying. Although in essence this is a "diet" designed to maintain your weight, if you're overweight you're likely to drop pounds. If you've reached a point where you're ready to be serious about your health and nutrition, you'll try to drink two quarts of water a day, and fit in a three to four day a week exercise regimen, too (more on that in Chapter 6).

◆

I personally also find that vitamin supplements are a good idea, because the fact is that no matter how hard we try, it's just not always possible to get all of what our bodies need from the foods we eat every day. I consulted JoAnn Smith, a nutritionist at Healthy Image in Los Angeles, and she suggests a multiple vitamin, a super-B complex, vitamin C (1,000 mg.), vitamin E (400 i.u.), beta-carotene (10,000 to 20,000 units), and for women over forty, calcium (900 mg.), plus zinc and magnesium.

◆

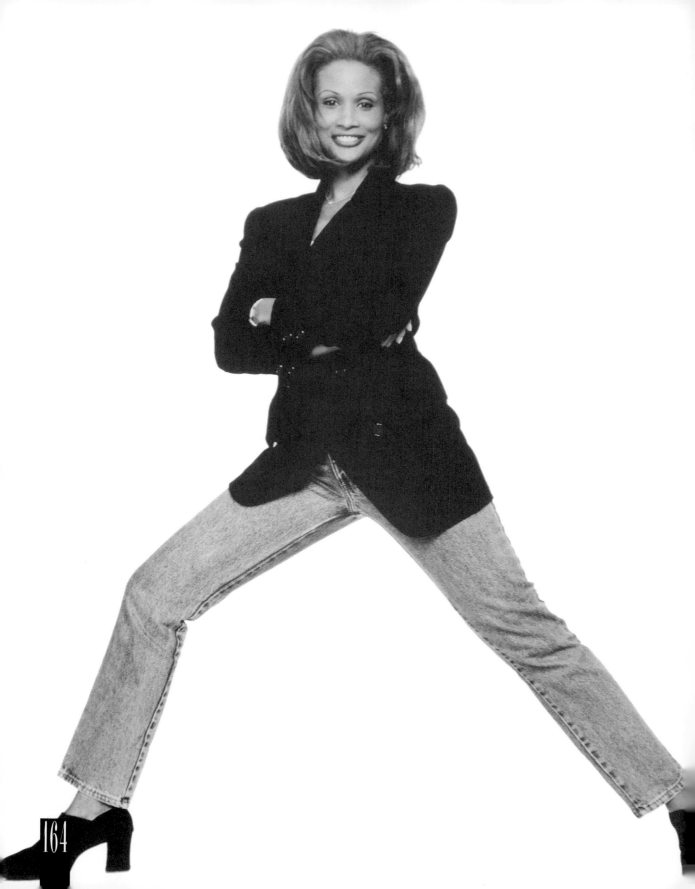

164

and a little pepper), one three-minute egg, and a glass of orange juice, or half a grapefruit or melon. If you don't care for orange juice you might create a mix of juices like apple, grapefruit, and orange. Or, instead of eggs and grits, try a bowl of bran cereal (like Wheaties or Raisin Bran), with a half cup of low-fat milk. But, whatever you do, don't skip breakfast.

Step 2: Around mid-morning a snack might be in order, depending on how hard I'm working or what's going on in my life. I might snack on an apple, some sunflower seeds, or my favorite, cut-up vegetables: celery, broccoli hearts, carrots, which I always carry with me in a little baggie (along with a bottle of ready-made, low-fat ranch dressing for dipping). It's amazing how having something like this on hand can save you from running to a vending machine or corner convenience store and grabbing a candy bar or a sugary soda.

Step 3: When I can, I like to start lunch with a big salad—iceberg or romaine lettuce, sliced tomatoes, the works, with low-fat dressing. If you make your salad big and substantial, you can actually fool yourself into thinking you're full. Follow up a modest salad with a half order of pasta: ziti or spaghetti or whatever your favorite is (remember, it's not the pasta but what you put on it—butter, cheese, loads of oily sauce— that's fattening). Good choices: cut-up vegetables; pesto sauce—a little, not a lot; Paul Newman's spaghetti sauce. My favorite is a pat of margarine, 1/4 cup of low-fat milk, a squeeze of lemon, and a sprinkle of parmesan cheese. For a change, try a cold pasta mixed with water-packed tuna and low-fat mayonnaise.

I also recommend having your biggest meal in the afternoon (I know that this can be hard to do, but as far as your body is concerned, it makes the most sense). If I am going out to lunch, for example, I try to order broiled or grilled fish, or calves' liver with onions, or a small Caesar salad or salad Niçoise.

Step 4: If I've had pasta for lunch, for dinner I might serve broiled or grilled fish

The rewards of eating healthy: real energy that doesn't quit.

**RESTAURANT STRATEGIES:
A GOING-OUT GUIDE**

*Here are some restaurant strategies I
learned up at Canyon Ranch Spa, in Tucson,
Arizona.*

1. *If the portions are very large, just eat
   half. When you're through, ask the
   waiter to remove your plate so you
   won't be tempted to keep eating.*

2. *When choices are limited, push gravy,
   rich sauces, and toppings to the side.
   Remove the skin from chicken, trim
   visible fat from meats, and peel off deep-
   fried batters.*

3. *Don't hesitate to ask how foods are
   prepared. Request no salt or monosodium
   glutamate and a minimum of butter,
   margarine, or oil.*

4. *Avoid adding protein to protein, such as
   cheese in omelets or on hamburgers—it
   tends to mean extra fat and
   unnecessary calories. Choose vegetable
   or mushroom omelets, plain hamburgers,
   vegetable-topped pizza.*

with a baked potato and broccoli. Fish can be especially easy to make: Just sprinkle with a little salt and pepper, and the smallest bit of margarine, and broil for a few minutes on each side. (The Canadian Fisheries Council recommends cooking fish a total of ten minutes per inch, regardless of the cooking method; it's the safest way to make sure you don't overcook it. Just measure it at its thickest point.) You might also want to squeeze a little lemon juice on top before eating—it's a no-calorie way to intensify flavor.

I've come to know for a fact that nothing replaces your basic three meals.

Other nights Anansa and I do a wonderful vegetable sauté: broccoli (you might want to steam this separately to keep it crisp), onions, and mushrooms all stirred together with garlic, low-salt soy sauce, and a little margarine. We serve it over steamed brown rice. For a change, we sometimes add a few pieces of cut-up skinless chicken breast. It's delicious, and all well within the range of that basic healthy eating plan.

It's ironic that at the heart of the healthy eating I've finally come to accept is my mother's original nutritional advice while I was growing up. "If you eat three square meals a day," she told me, "you won't gain weight." While I may have my baggie of vegetables between meals (or sometimes a vegetable/carrot/wheatgrass juice or a protein drink), I've come to know for a fact that *nothing replaces your basic three meals.*

HEALTHY RESTAURANT CHOICES

Appetizers: Order clear broths, consommé, bouillon, fresh vegetables. Avoid creamy soups, tortilla chips, anything fried.

Meat, fish, poultry: Order roasted, baked, broiled, grilled, steamed, or poached. Avoid fried, sautéed, stewed, braised, creamed, and breaded entrées. Ask for gravy and sauce to be omitted or served on the side.

Sandwiches: Order lean meat, fish, poultry (especially turkey) on whole-grain breads. Choose mustard instead of mayonnaise, butter, or oil. Avoid club sandwiches and fillings made with mayonnaise or salad dressing.

Eggs: Order soft or hard boiled, poached, or baked. Avoid fried, creamed, or deviled.

Potatoes: Order mashed (without butter or milk), baked, boiled, roasted, or steamed. Avoid fried, creamed, au gratin, or scalloped. Instead of butter, sour cream, cheese, or bacon bits, add plain yogurt, horseradish, salsa, chives, pepper, or lemon juice.

Vegetables: Order stewed, steamed, boiled or baked, without butter. Avoid creamed, scalloped, au gratin, sautéed or fried.

Salads: Instead of with dressing, order with vinegar and lemon. Avoid coleslaw and salads made with dressing, and molded canned-fruit and gelatin salads.

Breads: Order whole-grain breads, rolls, and cereals. Avoid sweet rolls, nut breads, coffee or pound cake, and sweetened cereal.

Desserts: Order fresh fruit, berries, sorbet, frozen yogurt. Avoid puddings, pastries and frosted cakes. If you can't resist, share a dessert with someone.

Beverages: Order bottled water, low-fat milk, or fruit or vegetable juices. Drink coffee or tea in moderation. Avoid sugared sodas and diet sodas (I find they actually make me crave salty and sugary foods), milk shakes, and alcoholic beverages. I also find that although sugar substitutes in morning coffee or tea may taste good, they tend to trigger my taste for sweets and salts, and I try to cut them out whenever possible.

SURVIVING ETHNIC AND FAST-FOOD RESTAURANTS

Chinese: Avoid pork, sweet-and-sour dishes, dishes made with nuts, tempura, egg rolls, or anything fried. Do not add soy sauce at the table. Choose stir-fried vegetables and chicken, seafood and bean curd dishes, and steamed rice. Request no MSG, salt, or soy sauce.

French: Avoid rich sauces, pastry shells, duck, and red meat. Order vegetables prepared without butter or margarine, and with sauce on the side. Choose chicken or fish dishes and eat only half.

Italian: Avoid creamy or cheese sauces and toppings (such as parmigiana) or fried dishes. On pizza avoid sausage, pepperoni, hamburger, anchovies, and olives. Order chicken cacciatore, pasta primavera, manicotti, and pasta with light clam sauce or marinara.

Mexican: Avoid guacamole and sour cream toppings, as well as cheese, sour cream, or beef entrées and anything fried. Order chicken or bean entrées, chicken enchiladas, bean burritos, tacos, tostadas, or tamales.

Eating out in the city—so many choices—can be tough. One strategy: decide in advance what you're going to order and stick to it.

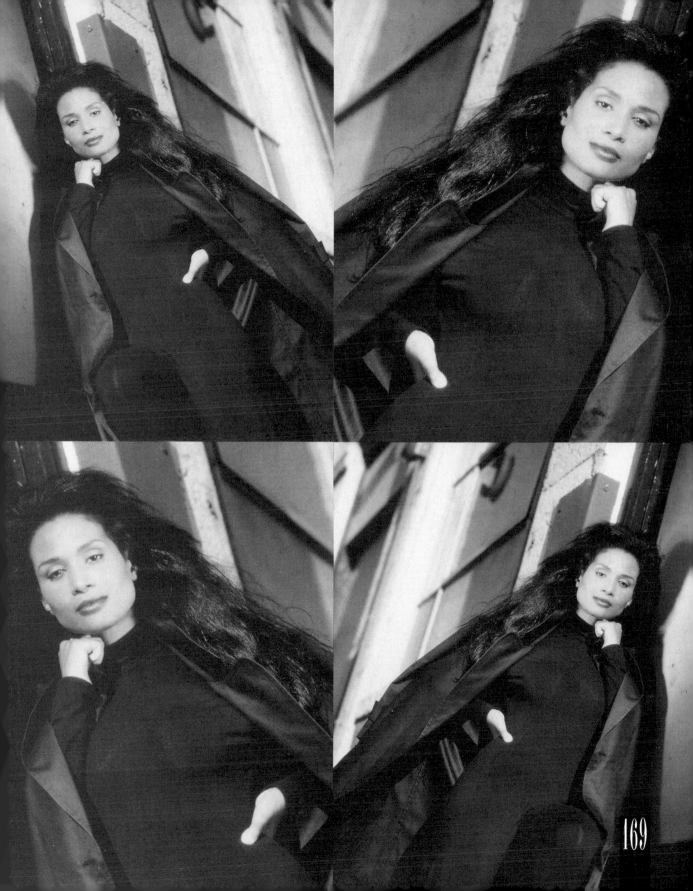

Salad bars: Avoid egg, cheese, meats, bacon bits, nuts, creamy dressings, potato and macaroni salads, and fried dishes. Choose fresh vegetables and greens with a few croutons and beans on top, and fresh fruit. Use lemon, vinegar, and pepper for dressing. If you order a chef salad, have the turkey, but skip the cheese, ham, and egg.

Delicatessens: Avoid salami, pastrami, corned beef and ham, and salads such as tuna, chicken, egg, and potato. Choose sliced turkey or chicken with mustard and assorted greens.

COPING STRATEGIES: FOODS TO ALWAYS HAVE IN THE HOUSE

I know that the idea of a lifetime plan may seem like a major commitment. Well, you're right, it is. But it's a commitment you're making to yourself and to reaching your own beauty and health potential. Still, until it becomes second nature, it can be hard to incorporate any new eating plan into one's life. To make it easier for myself (and, I hope, for you, too), here are some foods I always keep on hand:

Gallon-size containers of orange, apple, and grapefruit juice. Little half glasses of juice can be lifesavers, especially if you've got a sweet tooth. The next time you have the urge for something sweet, just drink 4 ounces of orange juice and it'll go away.

Gallon-size containers of water. Sometimes it's hard to

drink eight glasses of water a day, but you just do it (soon it will become the only thing that will quench your thirst). Besides helping to flush out your system, once you become attuned to your body signals, water will give you your second wind.

The idea of a lifetime plan may seem like a major commitment. But it's a commitment you're making to yourself and to reaching your own beauty and health potential.

Watermelon and other fruits, in season. Bagels and bagel chips. Non-fat yogurt in a nice variety of flavors (and in small sizes—just right for snacking, especially if you want something sweet late at night). Cereals, especially bran and wheat varieties. Saltine crackers (sometimes you just need something crunchy). Potatoes. Mustards, margarine, and lots of herbs and spices.

TIP

Diet tip: keep a food diary

One trick for monitoring my eating habits is to keep a food diary in which you write down every bit of food or drink—even if it's just a mouthful—that passes your lips. Try it for a week with a girlfriend, and I bet you'll be amazed at how easy it is to get amnesia about what goes into your mouth!

◆

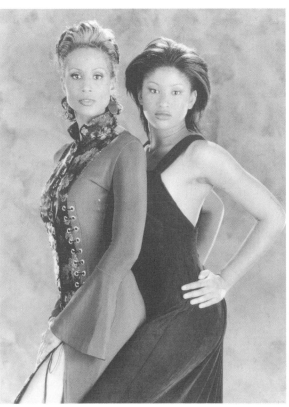

Healthy eating is easier when you have someone else to support you in your efforts. And, to applaud the results...

FAT, FOOD, AND DIET: UNDERSTANDING
THE NEW NUTRITIONAL PRIORITIES

One of the most important changes in nutritional advice in recent years is the emphasis on watching fat intake rather than calories. For those of us who grew up memorizing calorie charts, this new way of thinking has constituted something of a diet revolution. It's as if an entire generation's way of life (or way of eating) has vanished.

But there seems to be no question that the single most important dietary change you can make—to benefit your health and to control your weight—is to eat less fat, especially saturated fat. It's as simple as that. This is significant not only in terms of your appearance, but for your health's sake. Diets high in saturated fat promote heart disease, the disease the average person is most likely to die from.

Eat only in moderation—if at all—any foods containing more than four grams of fat per serving.

How this works: Saturated fat increases the amount of cholesterol in the blood, which gradually builds up in the arteries (much the way pipes in your kitchen sink can get clogged). Once an artery is blocked and blood is prevented from flowing to the heart, a heart attack can occur. In addition, high-fat diets in general have been linked to increased risk of breast cancer and cancer of the colon.

With all this in mind, how much fat should you eat? Probably the best rule for fat consumption is "the less the better." In fact, why not start by limiting yourself to a tablespoon of margarine a day, for example? I think you'll find that if you eliminate or reduce the fat from your diet, at the very least, you won't gain weight, and more likely, in the long run, you'll lose it.

"The more fat or saturated fat the food contains, the less of it you should eat," confirms the Center for Science in the Public Interest. According to the U.S.

Government's new "Dietary Guide-lines for Americans," a joint venture of the U.S. Department of Agri-culture and the Department of Health and Human Services, the average American should try to reduce his or her calories from fat to no more than 30 percent of daily total caloric intake. Other experts (including an independent panel put together by *Consumer Reports)* overwhelmingly favor cutting fat consumption further, advising that an adult's daily intake of fat should total no more than 20 to 25 percent of their total caloric intake. Of that figure, it's recommended that saturated fats should account for about 7 percent (or one-third total fat intake), with the rest comprised of unsaturated fat. Children over age two and teenagers are advised to consume up to 30 percent fat of their total caloric intake in fats (and up to 10 percent of that amount in saturated fats). Children under two should not have their fat intake restricted at all.

TIP

Saturated fat/unsaturated fat What's the difference?

Saturated fats, *which can be either animal or vegetable in origin, are the most dangerous. Most experts firmly believe that cutting back on saturated fats, which increase blood cholesterol, can significantly lessen your risk of heart disease. How do you know which fats are "saturated"? It's easy. Saturated fats are generally solid at room temperature and are found in fatty meats such as beef, pork, and lamb; in butter, whole milk, cheese and cream products; and in lard. It's important to remember that several kinds of vegetable oils are also highly saturated, namely coconut oil, palm kernel oil, and palm oil.*

◆

Unsaturated fats *consist of polyunsaturated fats and mono-unsaturated fats. Although it's best to avoid large quantities of any kind of fat, these are considered less harmful than those that are saturated. Unsaturated fats are liquid at room temperature: for example, vegetable oils, such as corn, soy, sunflower, and safflower are polyunsaturated. While these won't increase blood cholesterol levels the way saturated fats will, it's still somewhat controversial as to whether or not they can lower blood cholesterol levels. Mono-unsaturated fats may actually lower blood cholesterol levels and are considered by experts to be the best fats to consume in small quantities. Olive oil (considered one of the healthiest oils to use), canola oil, sesame oil, and peanut oil are all mono-unsaturated fats.*

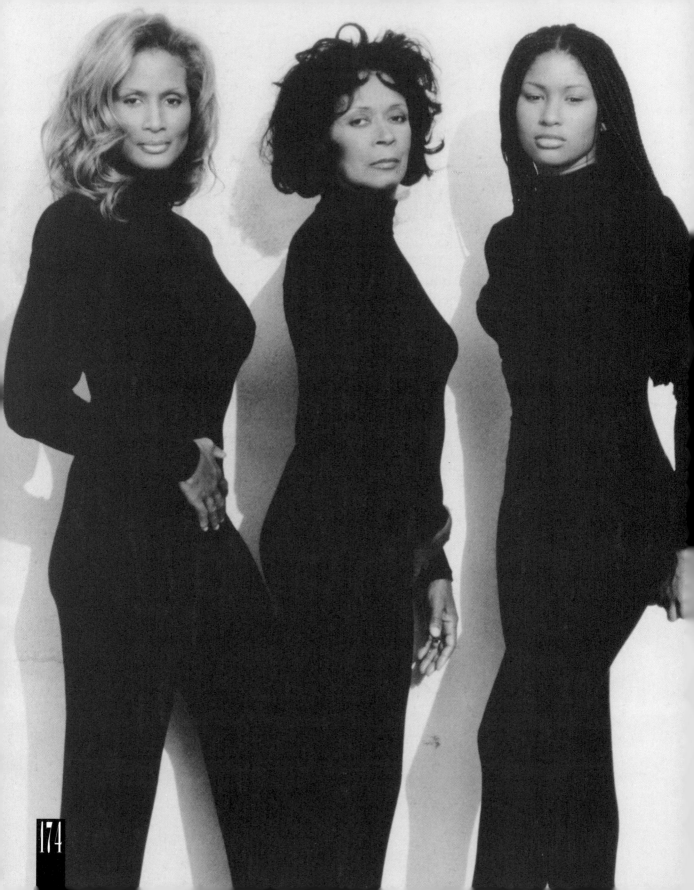

Fortunately, with so many people clamoring for lower-fat foods, literally thousands of low-fat or fat-free products are now on the market (nearly 1,000 new low-fat or fat-free food products were introduced in 1990 alone!). These include reduced-fat and fat-free ice creams, cheeses, and yogurts, low-fat crackers, cookies, soups, and salad dressings...even fast foods!

I do want to remind you that sometimes label claims of fat content can be misleading. For example, "lite" hot dogs, labeled 80 percent fat free, are actually less healthful than you would think, since 76 percent of their total calories are still derived from fat. The same goes for white meat chicken roll labeled 92 percent fat free; over half of its calories are from fat.

THE FOUR GRAM FAT RULE

If all this still seems confusing, here's an even simpler rule of thumb:

Eat only in moderation—if at all—any foods containing more than 4 grams of fat per serving.

Foods containing over 4 grams of fat tend to be over 30 percent fat, which is considered rather high. Although there are exceptions—some frozen dinners, for instance, have 8 fat grams and are only 27 percent fat—on the whole this is a safe and easy estimate to follow. To achieve this goal, try to substitute low-fat or fat-free foods for high-fat ones. For example, instead of frying in butter, oil, or margarine, fry in defatted chicken broth, water, wine, or any combination of the above. Low-fat cheeses

This picture—three generations—says it all: looking good isn't a matter of how old you are, but how fit you are.

HOW TO CALCULATE FAT PERCENTAGES

It's a good idea to know how to calculate fat percentages on your own. The following formula, based on 9 calories per gram of fat, is one that's widely recommended (I first learned about it at a health spa).

The percentage of calories derived from fat = grams of fat per serving X 9 divided by total calories from fat per serving X 100.

HOW IT WORKS:

1. Multiply total number of grams of fat per serving by 9 calories per gram. This gives you the number of calories from fat.

2. Divide the total number of calories from fat by the total calories per serving.

3. Multiply that number by 100. This figure is the fat percentage.

1 CUP LOW-FAT MILK

Calories: 120 per serving

Fat: 4.7 grams per serving

4.7 gms/serving x 9 calories/

gm = 42.3 calories from fat

42.3 calories divided by

120 calories X 100 = 35 % fat

175

are a good option. Instead of sour cream or butter on a baked potato, try low-fat ricotta cheese, non-fat plain yogurt, salsa, or mustard. For a low-fat pasta sauce, try sun-dried tomatoes (packed in water, not oil) blended in a food processor with a little water, a drop of olive oil, and garlic. Puréed prunes and a little cocoa powder can be an excellent substitute for butter in chocolate cake, because it has a creamy consistency and is sweet. Bananas or applesauce can also be used instead of butter or margarine in baked goods (for more healthy substitutions, see the boxed information opposite). And naturally it's a good idea to avoid deep-fried foods (which are breaded and fried), to trim the visible fat from meat before cooking, and to remove the skin from poultry.

Healthy eating is all about awareness.

Here are some additional substitutions to try (you might want to photocopy these pages and tape them on your pantry or refrigerator door):

On baked potatoes, try mustard, salsa, marinara sauce, non-fat plain yogurt, or non-fat cottage cheese.

On toast, bread or bagels, try sugar-free apple butter or sugar-free fruit spread, a tiny bit of honey and cinnamon, low-fat ricotta or non-fat cottage cheese.

On pasta, try marinara sauce; fat-free garlic-ranch dressing with parmesan cheese; non-fat cottage cheese blended finely with garlic and basil or garlic and roasted red or yellow peppers; 1/2 to 1 teaspoon olive oil with basil and tomatoes.

In tuna or chicken salad, try non-fat plain yogurt, with Dijon mustard and curry powder, fat-free mayonnaise, or fat-free ranch or other salad dressing.

Healthy eating is all about awareness. For example, Anansa and I try to stay away from fried foods as a rule. The other evening, though, I fried chicken for dinner and was so proud of the way it turned out. We may not serve it often, but when we do, we enjoy it. And even though I may enjoy it at the time, I also know—I'm aware—that that's not the way I want to eat all the time.

TIP

Healthy substitutions

Instead of	Try
Frying in oil, butter, or margarine	Frying in defatted chicken broth, water, wine, or any combination of these
Sour cream	Non-fat plain yogurt or non-fat sour cream
Cream cheese	Low-fat Ricotta cheese or blended non-fat cottage cheese or yogurt
Butter	Butter substitutes, plus cut the amount called for in half; in cookies use bananas or puréed prune
Cream or whole milk	Non-fat milk
Cheese	Low-fat cheese
Whole egg	2 egg whites
Sugar	Apple juice concentrate, fruit juices, applesauce, mashed bananas, puréed prunes
Salt	Lemon, garlic, onion, spices, herbs, salt-free seasonings

FOOD, FAT, AND YOUR FAMILY

My mother has made great strides getting my dad to eat vegetables and healthier foods, but the fact is that many women who are at home with young children or teenagers find it tempting to sample the ice cream and snack foods they feel they have to buy for their kids, or to join them in eating high-fat fast foods. The problem is that after eating this way the kids still stay skinny (most of them), but you get fat.

Getting in touch with your cravings

One of the strategies I've thought about is how to get from one meal to another, with only acceptable snacks in between. The key to doing this is to know which foods are your downfall. For example, I have a thing for sweets. I know that if I eat a candy bar, something inside me kicks in and I want another...and another. Try to identify what sort of foods trigger that uncontrollable response in you—then you'll know what areas to especially watch. This doesn't mean that you'll never be able to have those foods again. All it means is that this is a slippery area for you, and you need to be aware of it.

Solution: If you keep some of the foods on my healthy snack list in the house, you will always have the option of eating something different and not feeling deprived. Plus, because people all over are interested in eating well—and healthier—even fast-food restaurants these days offer choices such as salad bars and grilled (not fried) chicken sandwiches.

Remember, too, that children learn by example. By adopting healthier choices for yourself, you're not only showing your children that you care about your health, but you're serving as a role model for them as well. Try to improvise new low-fat ways of preparing your family's favorite dishes (use low-fat cottage cheese or low-fat Monterey Jack cheese on a baked potato instead of sour cream and bacon). Even a tiny bit of margarine goes a long way. The next time you're in a fast-food restaurant and tempted to steal one of your ten-year-old's french fries, just remember, it doesn't metabolize on him the same way it will on you!

FAT-FREE SNACK IDEAS

Air-popped popcorn, popcorn cakes, non-fat frozen yogurt. One-half baked potato with salsa, mustard, or fat-free plain yogurt. Bagel with sugar-free jam, jelly, or apple butter, salt-free pretzels. Steamed artichoke with lemon and mustard. Fresh vegetables and fresh fruit. Salads with diet dressing.

TIP ON WEIGHING IN

Experts suggest weighing yourself no more than once a week, because body weight normally fluctuates from one day to the next. Take your body measurements weekly—you may lose inches, not pounds.

SCALING DOWN

A food scale in the kitchen gets the message—and the reminder—across fast. Stock up on healthful foods—high in nutrients, low in calories and fats. That's the best way to "diet."

Not being hung up on that number on the scale...but still caring about healthy choices—there's a sense of freedom about getting to that point.

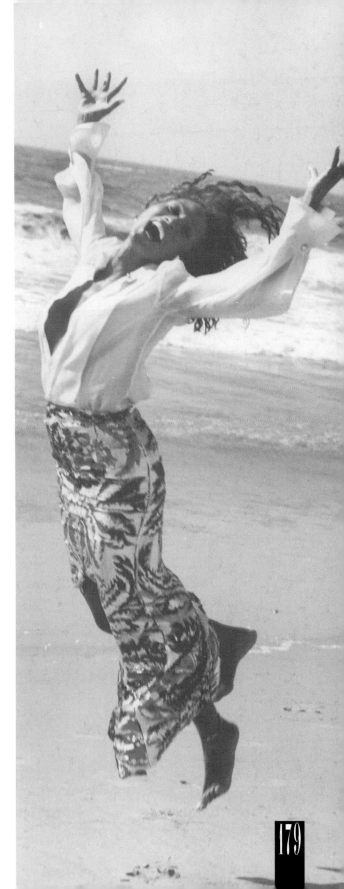

179

THE TEN POUNDS IN TEN DAYS HEADSTART PLAN

Should the loss of five or ten pounds boost one's self-esteem? In a perfect world, of course not. But in reality does it? Absolutely. Which is why I'm giving you my personal "Ten Pounds in Ten Days Diet"—the one I fall back on when I'm literally in a tight spot and have to drop ten pounds fast, for a movie, an important modeling job, a personal appearance.

Crash diets are not the answer. But we're all tempted to try one now and then. If you decide to give this one a whirl, just keep in mind that this is not a long-term eating plan for weight maintenance or weight loss. This is emergency treatment—when you need a quick boost to get you started or when you have to look good fast. Or use it for the allotted ten days only and with your doctor's permission, as a springboard into a sensible, everyday eating plan based on the ideas described in the earlier parts of this chapter.

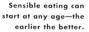

Sensible eating can start at any age—the earlier the better.

BREAKFAST:

1 protein serving (one 3–4 minute egg)

1 complex carbohydrate (one slice stone-ground toast)

Decaffeinated coffee or tea

(I also suggest starting the morning with a glass of water with lemon juice or a teaspoon of apple cider vinegar, in order to cleanse the system.)

LUNCH AND DINNER:

4 ounces of chicken or turkey, or 6–8 ounces of seafood

8 ounces (1 cup) vegetables or a salad of greens with lemon juice, 1 teaspoon virgin olive oil, and vinegar

(Three times a week, at either lunch or dinner, add 1 cup tofu or 1/2 cup pasta.)

SNACK:

1 piece of fruit

EATING DISORDERS

An eating disorder is actually a form of substance abuse in which food is the addictive substance. There are two common clinical conditions: anorexia nervosa, which is starving oneself thin (often combined with compulsive exercising), and bulimia, a syndrome of secretly bingeing on food, then purging via vomiting or laxatives. Both take the concept of "dying to be thin" to extremes and have killed thousands of young women either by malnutrition, heart disease, or kidney failure. Looking back, I'm lucky that I wasn't one of them.

Because of what I've been through with my weight, I'm particularly conscious of Anansa's attitudes toward food. Of course, I want her to be fit and healthy, but I'm also watchful that she doesn't fall into the same traps that I did. One time, for example, when

TIP

Basic ten-day rules:

1. Drink plenty of liquids throughout the day (at least 2 quarts). Herb tea, weak tea, distilled water, seltzer, and decaffeinated coffee are all allowed. No liquor or wine; no diet sodas, no juice.

♦

2. Salad dressing: 1 tablespoon virgin olive oil, vinegar, or lemon.

♦

3. No dairy products. No rice. Tofu in small amounts only.

♦

4. Ocean or sea salt in limited amounts.

♦

6. 1–2 lemons per day; seasonings and herbs allowed. One teaspoon virgin olive oil per day or one tablespoon for salad dressing.

♦

5. Pasta should be 100 percent semolina—1/2 cup, no more than three times a week.

6. Bread: 2–3 slices per day of stone-ground, seven-grain, or natural whole-grain breads (for example: for breakfast, 1/2 stone-ground English muffin; for lunch, stone-ground dinner roll; for dinner, Pritikin bread or pita bread).

♦

7. All protein must be unbreaded and boiled, broiled, baked, or grilled. No frying, no oils, except virgin olive oil. Small amounts of Pam may be used. Four ounces of turkey and chicken is one-half chicken breast or two legs or two small thighs. Remove all skin and visible fat before cooking.

♦

8. Fish or seafood (6–8 ounces at lunch and dinner). Choose from crab, lobster, shrimp, white fish, sole, perch, sea bass, halibut, snapper, salmon, trout, white water-packed tuna.

♦

9. Vegetables (8 ounces or 1 cup for lunch and dinner). Choose from asparagus, beet greens, broccoli, Brussels sprouts, cabbage, celery, chard, cucumber, kale, mustard greens, zucchini, lettuce, mushrooms, onions, radishes, spinach, green beans, tomato (1 small).

♦

we were taking a plane from Los Angeles to New York, and she was sitting in the seat behind me, I heard her tell the flight attendent who was serving the meal that she wasn't going to be eating (today she admits that, anticipating a modeling career, she was indeed trying to skip a meal). "Anansa, if you skip dinner, you'll be so ravenous tomorrow morning you'll end up eating two meals and more besides," I told her. It turned into a real tug of war, but in the end she understood—if begrudgingly.

Compulsive overeating, while not a textbook term, refers to a disorder in which an uncontrollable urge for food results in shame, self-hatred, and the disruption of the normal, everyday routines of one's life.

There are many possible causes for eating disorders such as these. One, of course, is the "thin ideal" adopted by our society. Another is distorted body image (in a study involving 1,000 pre-adolescent children, for example, 42 percent thought they needed to lose weight).

TIP

...Ten-day rules:

10. Fruits (1 per day between meals). Choose from 1 apple, 1/4 cantaloupe, 1/2 grapefruit, 1 orange, 10–12 strawberries, 1/2 pint black berries or raspberries.

◆

11. Daily vitamins: 500 mg. B6; 1,000 mg. bio-flavenoids; 800 mg. calcium (with magnesium and zinc); guar gum tablets; psyllium powder or tablets.

◆

12. Sweetener: Saccharin or Succaryl are okay.

◆

No additions or substitutions. Don't exercise strenuously, although moderate walking is okay.

◆

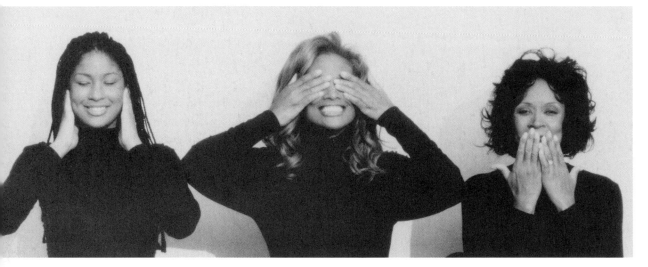

Hear no evil, see no evil, speak no evil. Closing your eyes to a problem won't make it go away.

But family or relationship problems can also trigger an eating disorder; so can stress in the form of never feeling good about oneself or feeling like an "impostor." People who are perfectionists—overachievers and obsessive types—may be particularly susceptible.

Are there any cures for these conditions? It depends. And treatment is a long-term and three-fold process.

The key thing is education. Young women with these conditions must be made aware of the terrible damage they are doing to their bodies. Books and magazine articles can help, as can visiting a bona fide nutritionist.

Behavior modification—for example, learning how to delay a binge or vomiting by writing in a journal or talking to a friend—is another method. This means trying to reeducate yourself and changing to a reality-based eating plan that consists of three meals a day (adding up to approximately 1200–1600 calories).

Finally, there's psychotherapy. Working with a therapist to build self-esteem, develop positive relationships, and learn coping strategies to deal with emotional highs and lows, pain and grief can help put food in perspective. (According to doctors, 80 percent of people with eating disorders are depressed.)

Can eating disorders be prevented? Perhaps not, but there are some things parents can do to help avoid them. First, help your children develop a healthy sense of self-esteem by becoming more conscious of the messages you give them. One study, for example, showed that in the course of a day, a teenager typically receives 400 negative comments versus 32 positive ones! When I read that I became even more conscious of how I speak to Anansa. Parents should also try to be aware of what's happening in school and in their child's general environment, and to "be there" for support. And set reasonable expectations for your kids; don't push for unrealistic goals and perfection.

Second, if you suspect a problem, call for help—a pediatrician, an internist, a therapist, or a clergyman.

Third, parents should strive to create goals for health within the family. Set an example of sensible eating; try to sit down with your family for at least one meal a day. Mealtimes, after all, are important family bonding times. And parents should try to control their own fanaticism about dieting and exercise. Kids, after all, are not deaf and blind.

♦

WHAT ARE THE WARNING SIGNS THAT PRECEDE AN EATING DISORDER?

Parents should not ignore these signs that their child might be in trouble:

- **Preoccupation with body image**
- **Fad or long-term dieting**
- **Use of diuretics or laxatives**
- **Weight loss without dieting**
- **Excusing oneself quickly during or after dinner**
- **Excessive exercise**
- **Depression or isolation**
- **Changes in behavior or self-esteem problems**
- **Excessive need for accomplishment**

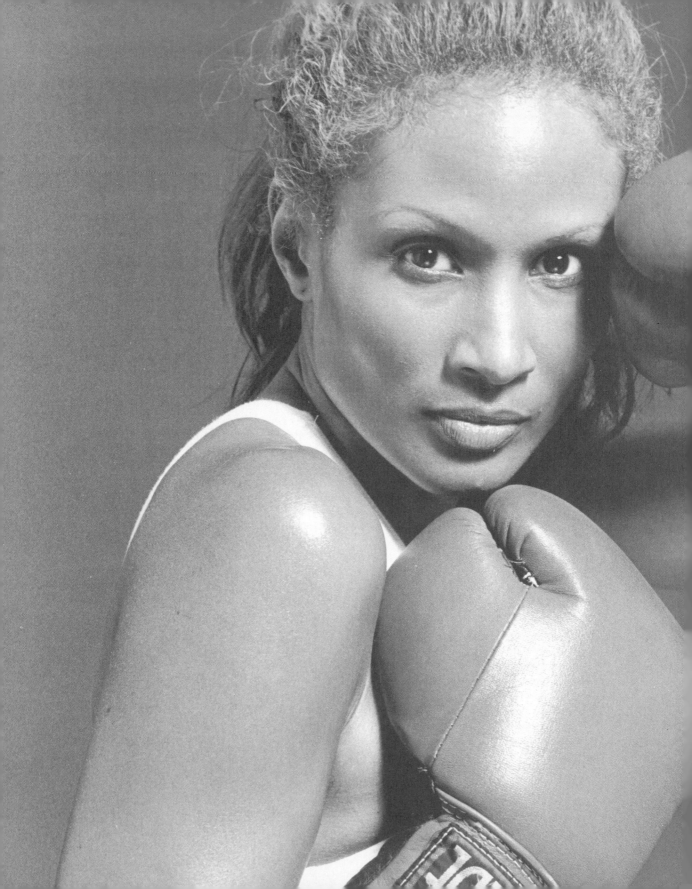

Chapter 6

True Beauty
Fitness

Strategies for the 90's

Fitness doesn't come from doing one particular kind of sport or exercise, but from a whole way of life. So what I want to talk about here is how to best incorporate exercise into your life—not necessarily so that you enjoy it (although that would be terrific), but, more important, so that you *do* it, especially if you've been resistant to exercising in the past or, like so many of us, simply can't find the motivation or the time.

First, understand that you are never too old, too young, or too out of shape to get started.

If you're reading this and you're in your teens or early twenties, you're smart and you're lucky. By taking the time now to learn about keeping your body fit, you're truly laying the groundwork for many positive years of beauty, health, and fitness. When you get in shape, and put fitness firmly in place in your life at an early stage, you'll be able to focus on more important goals—on completing your education, on getting your first job, on becoming independent and moving out on your own. The strength you gain will not only be physical, but psychological. You'll be one step ahead of the game.

Even though you may feel immortal now—perhaps you eat all you want without gaining an ounce or can slip into a bikini without giving sit-ups a thought—even though thoughts of wrinkles and sagging skin seem far, far in the future, keep in mind that the fitness habits you form early on have a lot to do with what's in store for you later on.

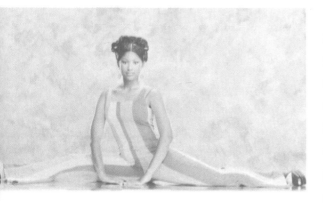

There's so much at stake. In addition to those physical activities you may already enjoy with your friends—whether it's going out dancing one or two nights a week, or playing a Saturday afternoon game of tennis or basketball—why not take the time to plan a basic fitness program you can maintain, at the very least a daily at-home program of aerobic exercise and some stretching? Although you probably care more at this point in your life about the visible effects on your tummy and thighs, it's the unseen benefits to your cardiovascular system (your heart and lungs) that will count most in the long run.

But what if you're young and overweight, as so many young women are. You may be surprised to hear me say that you're lucky, too. Because the body is an amazing, remarkable thing. If you make the effort to get fit now—if you decide now to embrace a life of healthy eating, of energy and activity—you have everything in the world ahead of you, all within reach. And while making a change in your life is never easy at any age, you've got time on your side. Get fit now while your body is young and at its most responsive, while your muscle tone can develop to its optimum. You're going to be able to experience real personal satisfaction, a special delight, as your body fat gradually disappears and your toned, firm, in-shape contours emerge. A good exercise program will keep you fit through the rest of your life, if you maintain and adapt it as your body changes.

AGE AND FITNESS

Even for those of us who make it a point to work to stay in the best shape we possibly can, there are inevitable changes in our body that come with age. Some I've accepted gracefully (at least I hope I have); others I've fought against (and I think I'm winning the fight—or at least keeping pace!).

Over 35. Typical trouble spots for many women over thirty-five include the upper arms, the stomach, and the waistline. For many women over thirty-five, in fact, a slight thickening of the waist, particularly after you've had children, is one of those almost inevitable body changes, and I always admire those women who keep their tiny waistlines as they get older. While my waist certainly isn't thick, it is an inch or two wider than it used to be. Just the other day, I was looking at Anansa's supple little waistline and remembering when mine was like that with practically no effort at all.

You can compensate for these changes by adding extra toning exercises and sit-ups to your regular exercise program, which is what I've done. I also stay in shape by consciously tucking in my stomach and holding it in at different times of day. At the same time, I've also noticed that my legs are better—stronger, shapelier and firmer—than they were when I was younger.

It's true, though, that as you enter your thirties or your forties, even if you've kept in

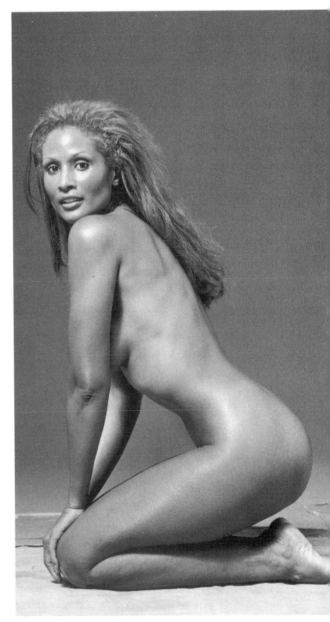

This photo was taken just a few months ago. As I've gotten older, I've added extra toning exercises (and especially sit-ups) in order to stay in shape.

189

good shape, you may notice that extra pounds or unwanted bulges just seem to appear more quickly than they did years ago, and are harder to get rid of, too. One of the reasons may be that our lives seem to become more sedentary. And that's where the importance of exercise comes in.

At this point, make an effort to be aware of your body's subtle (and sometimes not so subtle) changes: for example, a slightly thickening waist or a heavier upper arm. Listen to the messages your body is sending you and act on them. You may need to decrease your food intake in order to stay at the weight you want to maintain; you may certainly need to begin (or get back to) exercising regularly.

What so many of us seem to forget is that exercise is the reason that some women manage to maintain their weight, while others backslide. If you stay active—and this can mean as little as calisthenics for twenty minutes a day—you simply stand a better chance of staying in shape.

That's why exercise is more of an imperative than ever before (especially now, when your confidence about yourself should be at its peak). **To do:** Take the stairs instead of the elevator; walk whenever possible (instead of hopping in the car, on a subway, bus, or in a taxi). Join an exercise class—and enjoy the challenge.

As we get older, we do tend to be more sedentary, when it's really a time to step up activity. How about jogging?

Check out local health clubs (while some may be costly, many are surprisingly reasonable). Get a girlfriend (or your daughter, sister, boyfriend, husband, or "significant other") to join you. If you used to like to ride a bike, go back to it; if you think you may enjoy jogging or running, invest in a good pair of running shoes so you have a better chance of sticking with it. It's also important at this age to include exercises that relax you, that relieve stress, as well as those that tone your muscles, rev up your system, and get your heart rate going. Especially if the only time you have to exercise is at night, follow your workout with a soothing bath; otherwise, you may not be able to get to sleep.

Over 50. If you're in your fifties, sixties or seventies, don't fall into the trap of thinking that this kind of physical activity is over for you. The fact is that exercise is as important now as it was when you were younger. Aging occurs at different times to different degrees in all of us. With good habits—mental, physical, emotional—and good genes, you may even be feeling and looking younger than you have in years. You may be moving into a period where you have time, inclination, and knowledge that you didn't have before, and thus can be in better shape than ever.

Even though many experts find that women of color tend to have overall better muscle tone than other races, and to age more slowly, a certain loss of muscle tone and shifting of your body fat are going to be inevitable as you get older. While the right exercise program can't eliminate these changes, it can reduce them. But you may be experiencing other physical changes, too, such as varicose veins or slightly higher blood pressure, which will certainly affect the activities you can engage in. Your doctor, as well as your own body awareness and self-knowledge, will help you decide which movements and activities you want to participate in, and which you want to avoid. For example, you may not feel comfortable putting on a leotard and working out in a gym. If so, that's fine. Of course, if you've always managed to stay fairly fit, you probably

Our landmark
photo, all
beauties of
color, this
page, clockwise
from the top:
Kara Young,
Cynthia Bailey,
Rashumba,
Gail O'Neil.
Opposite: me,
Beverly Peele,
Lana Ogilvie,
Louise Viette.

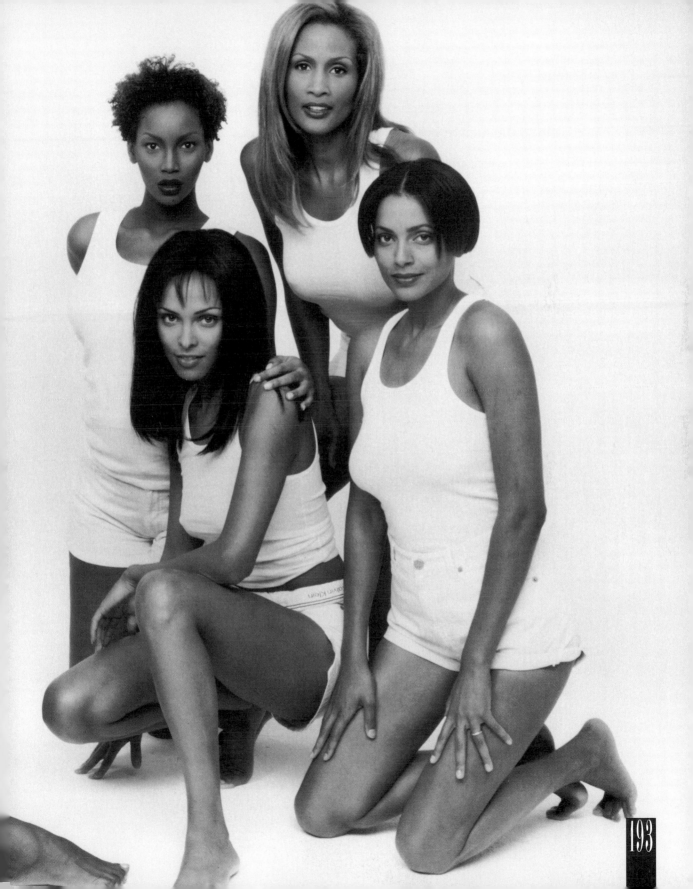

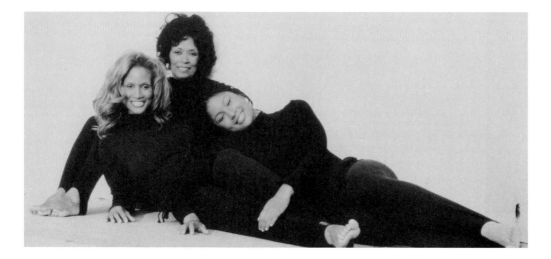

A family that exercises together, collapses together!

won't be experiencing as many of the effects of getting older as your contemporaries who haven't.

But it's also never too late. If you haven't exercised regularly while you were younger, if you're overweight and out of shape, you can start now, and feel younger and better about yourself as a result of it. Check it out with your doctor first, of course. If he or she approves, join an exercise class (with a teacher who is experienced in working with older women). An even simpler alternative: Get into walking (experts say that fast walking is one of the most effective aerobic exercises, at any age). Get a friend involved and plan on walking several miles a day, increasing the mileage as you both become more fit.

GETTING INTO A LIFETIME EXERCISE HABIT

One way to get into the exercise habit is to think of exercise not as an option, but as a given: something as routine as washing your face, brushing your teeth, or putting on your shoes in the morning. If you stop thinking of exercise as a luxury and start regarding it as a necessity—for your looks, for your health—while you won't necessarily come to love it (although you certainly could), you will do it. Besides, getting into exercise can help you change your eating habits and attitudes toward food (one effort tends to fuel the other). Plus, exercise burns calories not only while you're doing it, but long after the activity has stopped, because it increases your metabolic rate as well.

Another way to accept exercising into your life is to find an exercise partner—a good friend, a sibling, your mother or your daughter, your mate. Take the time to figure out the type of exercise you would most enjoy doing, or at least would be able to tolerate. This can go a long way in determining whether you stick with an exercise program or drop out. For example, I tend to get terribly bored when I take a dance-oriented exercise class. Although I love to dance, I just don't seem to want to do it in a gym. Mind you, other people thrive on it—and get terrific results.

I've discovered I prefer to take my physical activity in active sports: biking, hiking, basketball, volleyball, roller-skating—all the things I loved to do as a teenager. And I like to make it a family affair, too, something we all can do together. For instance, Anansa and I enjoy renting bikes on a Sunday afternoon and exploring the biking trails nearby.

But as much as I try to incorporate the sports that I love into my life, I also realize that sports activities alone don't constitute a good workout. That's because many sports such as tennis or basketball are usually "stop and start" activities and don't provide substantial aerobic benefits (swimming, on the other hand, does). Second, if you don't work out to prepare yourself for sports, you could end up with an injury. That's why I make it a point to stretch every day, to take body sculpting classes when I can, to work out with a trainer. I also strongly believe in varying my exercise from time to time, to avoid the kind of monotony that statistics say causes so many

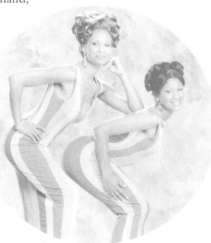

Have a buddy when you excercise— Anansa is mine.

TIP

Exercise safety tips

Check with your physician before beginning any exercise program.

◆

Keep your head up to avoid dizziness.

◆

Work at your own pace. Don't push yourself. Stop if you need to, and drink water to stay hydrated.

◆

Don't bounce when you stretch.

◆

Listen to your body. If you feel sore, stiff, or tingly, give yourself a day off from exercise.

◆

people to drop out. Recently, for example, I've been on a running kick: I get up at 5:30 every morning, meet a friend and we run five or six miles—and I feel charged and energized for the rest of the day.

Other ways to keep fitness and exercise a vital part of your life, all your life? Consider a fitness-oriented vacation, where you're active and on the go—going to a riding ranch, going hiking or trail-walking, skiing, or especially to a spa or health resort. For me, this is the ideal getaway—the chance to assess where you are mentally, physically, emotionally, and even spiritually, and where fitness takes on a new dimension. At a spa, the only things you have to do are pamper yourself, eat healthy, low-fat meals, and work out. It's a great way to concentrate on self-improvement, body and soul, without the intrusion of outside anxieties and responsibilities. And there are so many these days, in a surprisingly wide range of prices, from budget to deluxe, and in a wide range of styles, from ultra-Spartan to ultra-luxurious. A spa is a great place to take those first steps to personal achievement, to striving to do or be the very best at what is important to you—whether that's building a beautiful home, being the best parent or the best spouse, rising to the top of your class, or becoming the most creative or most outstanding at your job. To do any of these things—and more—it's absolutely essential that you take care of yourself first; otherwise, you're not going to be able to go the distance.

EXERCISES FOR GETTING FIT AND STAYING FIT

Exercise can either relax you or invigorate you, depending on the type of activity you do. Aerobic exercise such as running, fast walking, or a fast game of tennis, gets oxygen into your blood, reviving you and making you feel more energetic and awake (that's why, if you plan your aerobic workout too late in the day, you may find it harder to fall asleep). Stretching, strengthening, and calisthenics do just the reverse, producing a fatigue response in muscles.

In order to be fit, everyone, whatever her age or race, needs to incorporate three kinds of activity into her exercise plan:

• Strengthening exercises, which increase the strength of muscles via weight machines or calisthenics (such as push-ups or sit-ups) or weigh-training exercises.

• Endurance exercises, which consists of aerobics for cardiovascular health. For best results, these activities should be done at your target rate—the highest rate of intensity you can do continuously—for at least twenty minutes. Aerobic exercises include walking, jogging, biking, running, aerobic dancing, step aerobics, swimming, jumping rope, rowing, calisthenics, and machine workouts such as the treadmill or the Lifecycle or Stairmaster.

• Flexibility exercises, which lengthen muscles through stretching movements.

To see fitness benefits, a workout including these three elements should be done at least three times a week. In addition, African-American women should make a

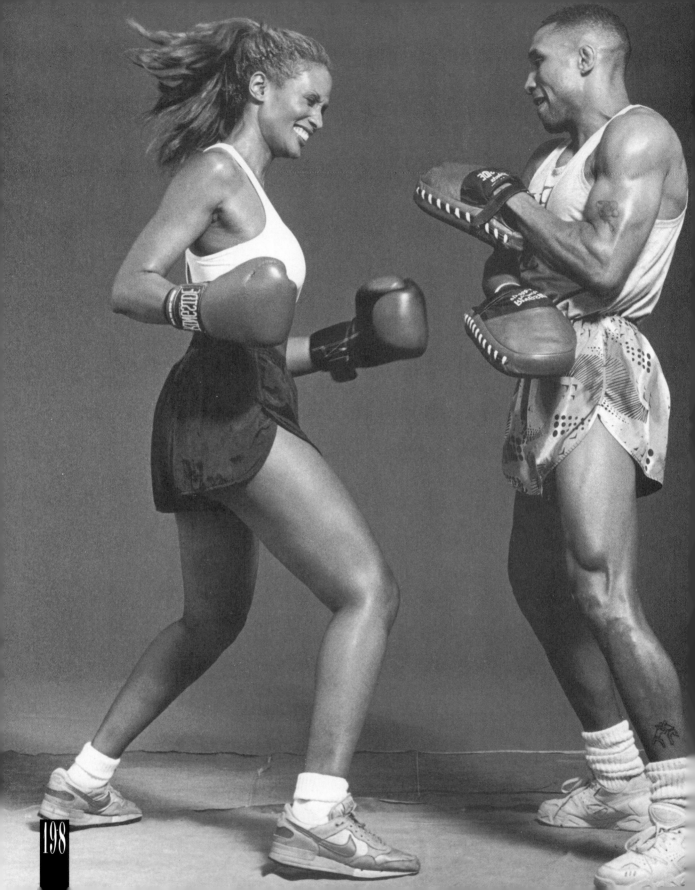

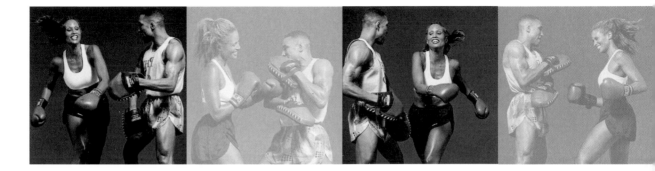

special effort to include abdominal-strengthening, foot-strengthening, and knee-balancing exercises to compensate for the increased angle in their lumbar spines.

How long should your workout last? About twenty-five to thirty-five minutes per session, about three times a week, is currently accepted as ideal. It's all very well for some celebrities to brag about spending three to five hours a day working out to get in shape for a special role, but that's hardly realistic for anybody else. If you manage to stick with a twenty-five to thirty-five minute workout, three times a week, and combine it with a low-fat eating plan, you'll lose weight—slowly, perhaps, but you will.

FREQUENTLY ASKED QUESTIONS ABOUT FITNESS

Q. What happens to a woman of color's body as she ages?

A. Most women (and men) have a tendency to become flabbier, put on weight, and "spread" with age. Luckily for African-American women, our higher bone density helps protect us from the onset of osteoporosis. And our skin elasticity helps us stay firmer longer. On the negative side, stretch marks from pregnancy or weight gain do tend to look more pronounced on darker skin. As a black woman ages (say, between forty-five and sixty-five) her breasts may drop, her triceps and inner thighs may get wiggly, but her buttocks will stay high.

Boxercise—it relieves tension, burns calories and it's fun.

Q. What's the best exercise plan for lifetime fitness?

A. According to fitness experts, one that's based on strength, endurance, and flexibility activities. And it's never too soon to start. Fortunately, young girls and teens have mandatory gym classes (which have dramatically changed since I was in school). Now the emphasis is on creating body awareness and developing a total fitness program early on. Also, thank goodness, we've started to realize that being strong and fit is no longer just a boy's thing. Many girls have come to recognize that proficiency in sports can lead to fame and fortune (think of college scholarships and FloJo).

In mid-life, it's important to continue with an at-least-three-times-a-week fitness plan. Hopefully these are the years when a woman will be more in tune with herself and her body. By now, you should know that your best exercise regimen consists of something you like (or at least don't hate), and that it is affordable and convenient. This may be the time to make an appointment with a trainer to develop a quality workout. Remember, it's not the amount of time a workout takes, but how efficiently it works and if you stick to it.

Plus, as a woman gets older, she needs to do more—not less—exercise, although it certainly may be at a lower intensity, such as yoga. As long as you're in good health, it's important to keep up your commitment and involvement to stay vital. Never use aging as an excuse. Keeping active is good for one's heart, one's mind, and especially one's self-esteem.

Q. What are the most efficient exercises a woman can do?

A. Actually, you shouldn't do the same workout every day because your body needs a day off to repair and build. This means you should alternate the muscle groups you work on. For example: one day, concentrate on the upper body; the next, on the lower. And, for variety, you might want to alternate your aerobic activities, too.

I'm not a great rider, but it's invigorating, tension-relieving (and it burns calories like crazy).

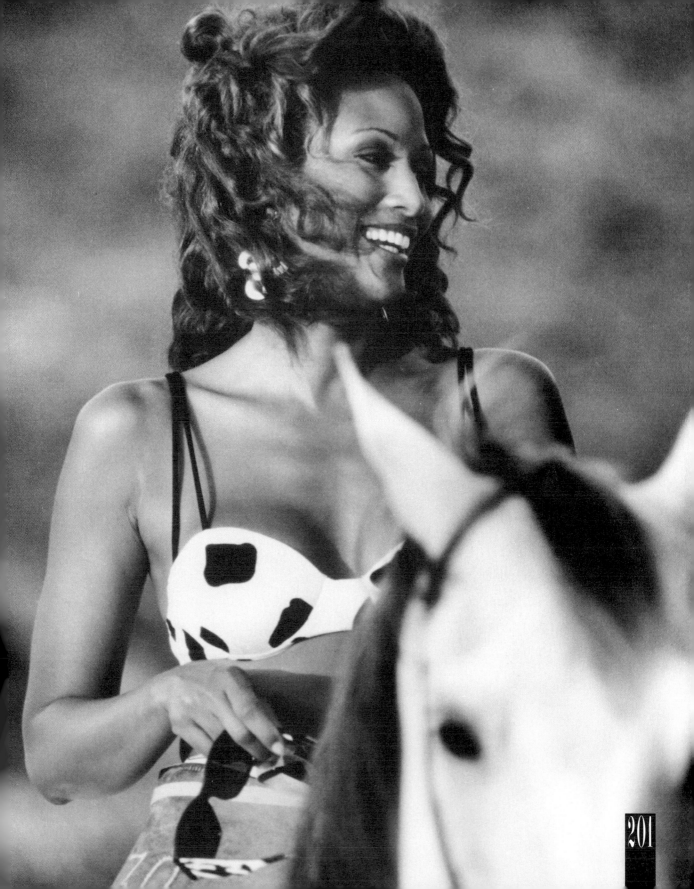

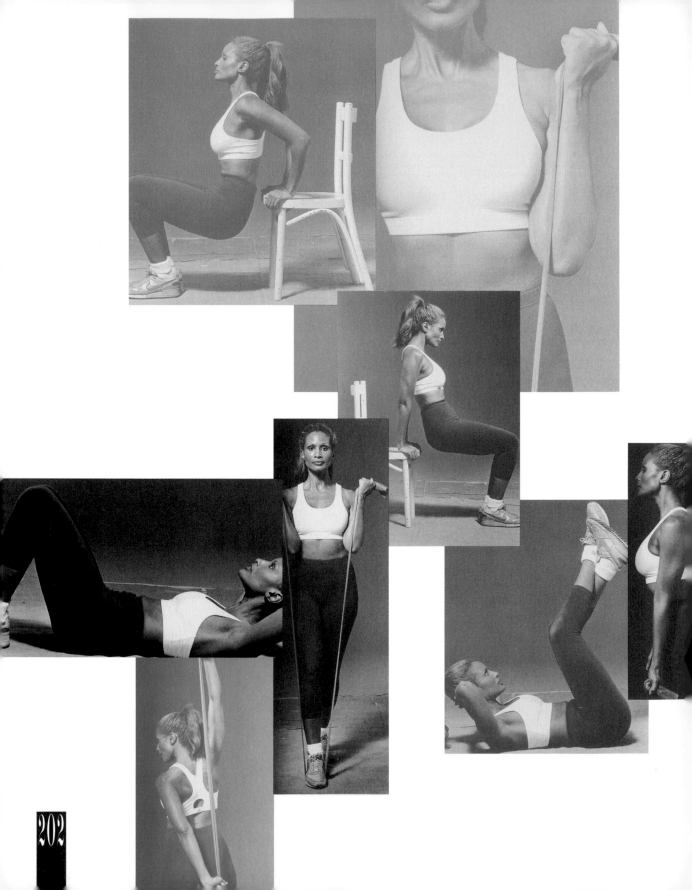

Here's a sample menu of top trainer-recommended exercises:

FOR YOUR UPPER BODY

Push-ups. Beginners may need to begin from a standing position, using resistance from the wall. The goal is to build up the strength to work from the floor—first with your knees on the floor (women's push-ups) and eventually men's push-ups, with your feet on the floor. Keeping your back and neck straight, tummy tucked, and elbows bent, exhale, and, straightening your arms, lift your body off the floor. Inhale as you lower. Begin with two sets of six repetitions; work up to four sets of eight.

Dynaband Workout. These long, resistant rubber "ropes" with handles do wonders! Available at sporting goods stores, they cost about $5. Use them for biceps curls (curling arms forward), triceps lifts (raising straight arms behind you), and lifting arms straight out at your sides. You can do the same with two- to five-pound dumbbells, but dynabands are much harder.

Triceps Presses. Sit on the floor, supporting yourself with arms behind you, fingers facing forward, and heels on the floor. Slowly lift your buttocks off the ground, bending your elbows as your butt touches the floor. Remember to keep your abdominal muscles tucked. Start with two sets of six repetitions; work up to four sets of eight.

FOR YOUR MIDDLE BODY

Sit-ups. Lie down with your feet on floor, knees bent, and hands resting lightly behind your neck for support. Slowly lift your shoulders off the ground, with your chin pointed to the ceiling. Exhale as you lift. Inhale and lower. (Do the same number of reps as for other exercises.) As you become stronger, lift yourself higher and tilt your pelvis. Remember to keep your abdominal muscles contracted.

Crunches. Lie on the floor with your knees lifted and your hands resting lightly behind your neck for support. Hold in your abdominal muscles, exhale, and crunch up, bringing your upper body toward your knees. Hold for three seconds, exhale and curl down to the floor. (Do the same number of reps as you do for other exercises.)

FOR YOUR LOWER BODY

Squats. (For buttocks and thighs.) Hold on to a chair for support. With your feet and knees facing forward, back straight, abdominal muscles contracted, and pelvis tilted, exhale and slowly lower yourself to a sitting position. Don't go all the way down; don't lock your legs or snap your knees. Slowly lift yourself up and repeat. (Same number of reps.)

Plies. (For buttocks and inner thighs.) A variation of a squat. Here your knees and feet face the sides. Keep your back flat, abdominal muscles tucked in, and neck straight. Carefully bend from the knees, making sure your kneecap is aligned with your foot. Squat only to a 90-degree angle. (Same number of reps.)

Lunges. Keeping your back straight, and abdominals and butt tucked under, place your right foot in front with your right leg slightly bent. Slowly lower your left knee toward the floor, then lift. Change legs and repeat. (Same number of reps.)

ANOTHER APPROACH: LIPOSUCTION

Liposuction, pronounced to rhyme with "typo," is the surgical removal of fat from localized parts of the body. How curious—and hopeful!—everyone always is about it. In truth, liposuction is an amazing process, but keep in mind that it's not a miracle cure by any means, nor is everyone eligible for it. Plus, not only is it expensive but a lot depends on finding exactly the right professional—one who is skilled and experienced at performing these operations, otherwise you'll end up with an ugly dimpled effect. With that said, here are some of the basic things you need to consider.

We all know that there are some areas of the body where fat deposits tend to accumulate that simply don't respond well to exercise or dieting, no matter how diligent you are or how hard you try. These hard-to-reduce areas can include the chin, cheeks, neck, upper arms, abdomen, upper-thigh area, hips, buttocks, and knees. For many African-American women and some Latin women in particular, the area that concerns us most is the tendency to heavier thighs—some people call them "saddle-bag thighs." So many women tell me how they hate the way their "saddle bags" look when they wear tight jeans or pants!

For some women, liposuction (also known as suction-assisted lipectomy) is the answer. In fact, although it's been performed in the United States only since 1982 (at which time it was greeted with tremendous skepticism by the medical establishment), in only ten years it's become *the* most commonly performed cosmetic surgical procedure for women today (and the third most popular for men), according to the American Society of Plastic and Reconstructive Surgeons. Of those women who elect liposuction, 39 percent are between the ages of thiry-five and fifty. As for price, surgeon's fees for the various liposuction techniques range from $500 to $5,000, with an average of $1,480.

Generally, liposuction has been successfully performed on the neck and chin areas, the lateral (outer) thighs (known as the "riding britches" or "saddle bag" area), the abdomen, and the inside of the knees. Less commonly, it's also performed on the ankles and calves. When it's done well, while it's not a cure-all (you can only remove about two pounds of fat at a time), it can help you feel better, look better, and fit better into your clothing. In short, it can help you feel much more attractive.

How does liposuction work? The procedure involves the use of a hollow metal tube or pipe (called a canula) that is attached to a powerful suction machine. The canula is inserted into the body through a small incision and manipulated deep within the fat layers under the skin. As it's moved back and forth, it breaks up the fat globules, actually suctioning them out.

ETHNIC WOMEN AND EXERCISE

If you make a study of body types and fitness, you'll find that there are differences among the races that are generally acknowledged by physicians and fitness experts alike. Some of these differences, which I learned from my doctor and my trainer, may surprise you, some may intrigue you, but all of them can be helpful, when you start to consider your options in terms of getting and staying fit.

While no two people are exactly alike, similar ethnic groups do share certain characteristics. According to experts, African-American women in general tend to have better muscle tone than white women. Whereas white women may carry weight in their hips, stomach, and inner thighs—and have a tendency to develop fatty dimples at the backs and sides of their upper thighs and on the buttocks (as well as to develop fleshy upper arms in later life), black women are naturally firmer overall. Traditionally we tend to have large, yet firm, high and "perky" buttocks, and large muscular thighs (flabby thighs aren't usually a problem for African-American women unless they're very heavy). Younger black women usually have slim torsos, flat abdominal muscles, and rather toned triceps.

When the procedure was first pioneered, a fairly large canula, sometimes as large as one-half inch in diameter, was used. This tended to leave surface imperfections and irregularities. Today more experienced surgeons and smaller canulas (one used for the neck might be as tiny as 2 millimeters in diameter) have resulted in vast improvements. This smaller canula may require more back-and-forth motion, but it also results in a much smoother surface.

I have to admit that many people in the modeling business have liposuction when they don't really need to (a lot of people look at it as an easy way to lose weight, which it is most emphatically not). However, there are sometimes tough areas where it is nearly impossible for you to eliminate fat through dieting and exercise. I personally think that under the right circumstances, and if you can afford it, liposuction is worth a try, if you understand all the risks that are involved.

If you are seriously considering liposuction, you should realize that the results are dependent not only on what you remove, but on what you leave behind to maintain the surface smoothness of your skin. For example, you're certainly not going to remove *all* the fat from a given area, because that won't create a normal appearance. Plus, I have to repeat that, despite its tempting success rate, liposuction should not be regarded lightly or considered as an alternative to weight loss. It is surgery, make no mistake about that. And because it works best when the problem is localized—removing distinct fat bulges that are disproportionate to the rest of the body and are non-responsive to diet and exercise—it's not for someone with a generalized problem (someone who is extremely overweight or someone who has heavy thighs all around).

In addition, there's a limit to how much fat you can remove at one time without requiring a blood transfusion. Because fat loss is accompanied by blood loss, liposuction can remove only about two pounds of fat at one time. In some instances, however, suctioning of larger amounts of fat is possible if the patient donates blood in advance. But it's not the way to lose twenty pounds fast!

Other points to know: Good skin tone is essential for best results. If your skin is flabby or loose, liposuction is *not* the answer. When the skin tone is good, however, a tremendous improvement can be obtained by the suctioning of excess fat. Plus, as long as you maintain a weight within the range of your weight at the time of surgery, the fat should not come back and the procedure should not have to be redone.

What about scarring—a matter of special importance to African-Americans? Fortunately, it's generally minimal, since only extremely tiny incisions that are generally hidden in body creases are necessary. Because of the tininess of these incisions, even if you're prone to keloids they are likely to be very small.

After a lipectomy, you can generally expect to be back to work within one to two weeks, and able to take on strenuous activity within two to four weeks, although swelling and bruising can last from one to six months or more. If you have it done on the abdomen, you will probably have to wear some kind of pressure binder (such as a surgical girdle or elastic dressing) continuously for about a week to minimize bruising and swelling, followed by two to three weeks of wearing it just during the day, for additional support while your body assumes its new shape.

◆

African-American women also tend to have an increased angle in the lumbar spine. This is actually thought to be a result of our native heritage, going back to the days when our ancestors walked barefoot, carrying heavy objects on their heads. Today, I've been told, it's important to know about this inborn condition because it actually can affect body mechanics, contributing to weaker abdominal muscles and a higher incidence of fallen arches and hyperextended knees.

To compensate for the increased angle in the lumbar spine, specially directed exercises may be in order. We may need to especially focus on abdominal strengthening exercises (such as modified sit-ups), foot-strengthening exercises (such as heel raises and toe pointing and flexing), and a variety of leg exercises to "balance" hyperextended knees. Luckily African-Americans also seem to have higher bone density, which makes us less prone to osteoporosis in later life and more likely to have better posture.

Latin women fall somewhere between African-Americans and Caucasians. My Latin friends describe their typical body type as medium-muscled, often with thickish legs, strong calves, and high, wide rear ends. Usually on the short side, Latin women can appear chunky in later life if they don't work out.

For women of color, they tend to appear almost delicate by comparison.

207

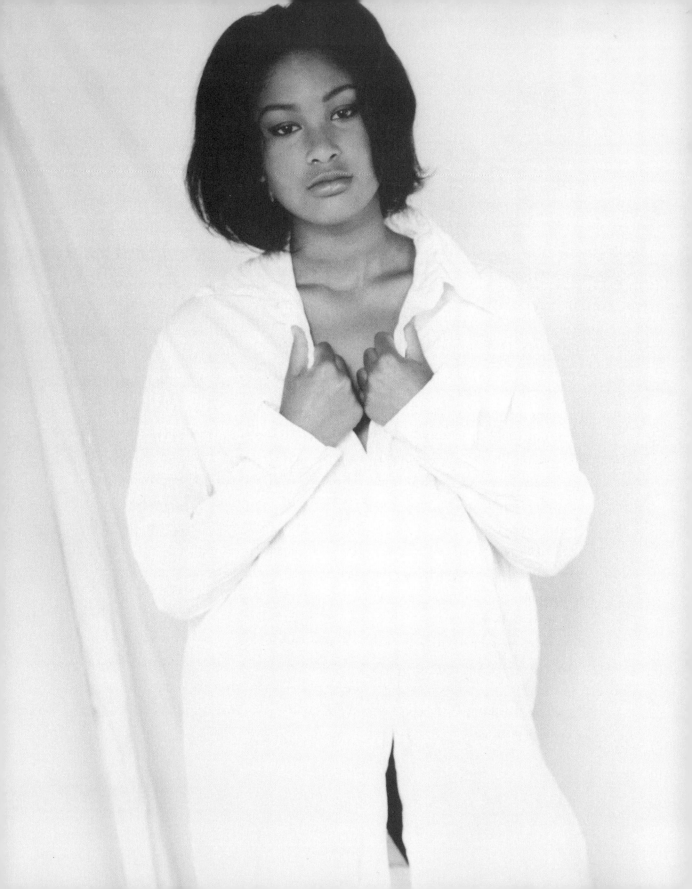

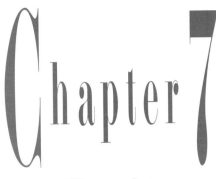

Chapter 7

Thoughts on Your Well-Being

The Link Between Mind and Body

True Beauty. All of the makeup tools and techniques, all of the hair-care advice, all of the fitness and nutrition pointers I've gone through in the preceding chapters are only part of the story. That's because the real secret of true beauty is dependent on your emotional and spiritual well-being as much as your physical attributes.

Having focused on the physical issues, if you're now ready to tackle the final step—to put your energy into making those changes that will truly enhance the quality and, yes, the beauty of your life—read on. Of course, a major part of beauty is physical: No one is denying that. Taking quality care of your skin and hair, learning to eat well and healthily, to dress with ease and simplicity, to develop and maintain a sense of your own personal style—these are certainly steps in the right direction. In fact, they may be as far as you're ready to go for now. If so, that's fine.

But if you're ready to go further, know that the link between mind and body is a vital one—and one that's well worth exploring. For example, no one questions that hormones can affect your mood, your energy level, your appetite. Personal stress and anxiety—the loss of a loved one; disappointment in a relationship; trouble with a child, a parent, a spouse, a job—all of these tensions can take their toll on your looks, body, and mind.

You may be ready to accept some of the ideas and therapies I'm going to be discussing in the pages ahead; others you may reject, or perhaps come back to at another point in your life. What I hope, though, is that you'll be interested enough to explore, open enough to reach out, and sufficiently ready to recognize that this route is indeed the secret, the key, the heart of true beauty, inside and out. The common ground of these methods is that they are all directed to making you feel positive about yourself, to making you know that you are worth the effort.

UNDERSTANDING SOUL-ESTEEM: WHAT IT IS, WHY YOU NEED IT, HOW TO GET IT

Of course, you've probably realized that a good deal of what I'm talking about is based on simple self-esteem. As much as the tides of the lives of women have turned generally for the better, the lack of appreciation of our own self-worth and power remains a critical factor in our lives. However, it's not only self-esteem that counts, but also what I like to distinguish as soul-esteem.

Soul-esteem has less to do with rigid (and ultimately self-defeating!) exercises in self-control than with self-development. And it's from the development and nurturing of your own psychological and spiritual base—in which you allow yourself to take time to sit quietly, to be still and tap into your own intuitive self—that the nurturing of your essential soul-esteem begins.

Now, there's no need to tell me that you don't have time to do this. I know that.

Few of us do. That's the problem, and it's very much a modern-day phenomenon. Society has placed us as women of color—as women in general—into a giving position. We're always caring for others, whether it's our spouses, our children, our families, our friends, our jobs, or our homes. But there comes a time when you just become so tired, so fatigued, both physically and emotionally, that you can't go on. That's when you need to take the time to give back to yourself—to stop and gather your inner forces and replenish your soul.

Perhaps you feel you just can't do this—or you don't know how to begin. Perhaps you feel as if you're dealing with a crushing number of demands and expectations, that you are being called upon to "be perfect" in every aspect of your life (to be a perfect mother, perfect wife, perfect friend, perfect cook or homemaker, perfect employee). But as you try to do your best in every area (from your work to your exercise routine!), to truly live a life of beauty, you must make time to nurture your inner self. It's this and only this that makes it possible to continue. This is what forges us, what enables us to do everything else.

Perhaps, though, you feel you don't even have that fundamental inner core I'm talking about

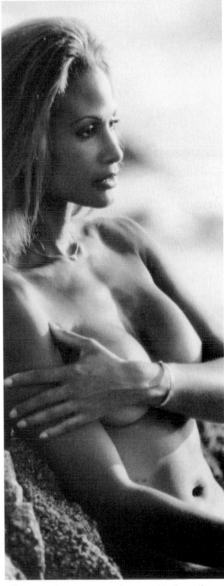

When you strip away externals, you get to the real you...and it's what's inside—the beauty of the spiritual, emotional you—that really counts.

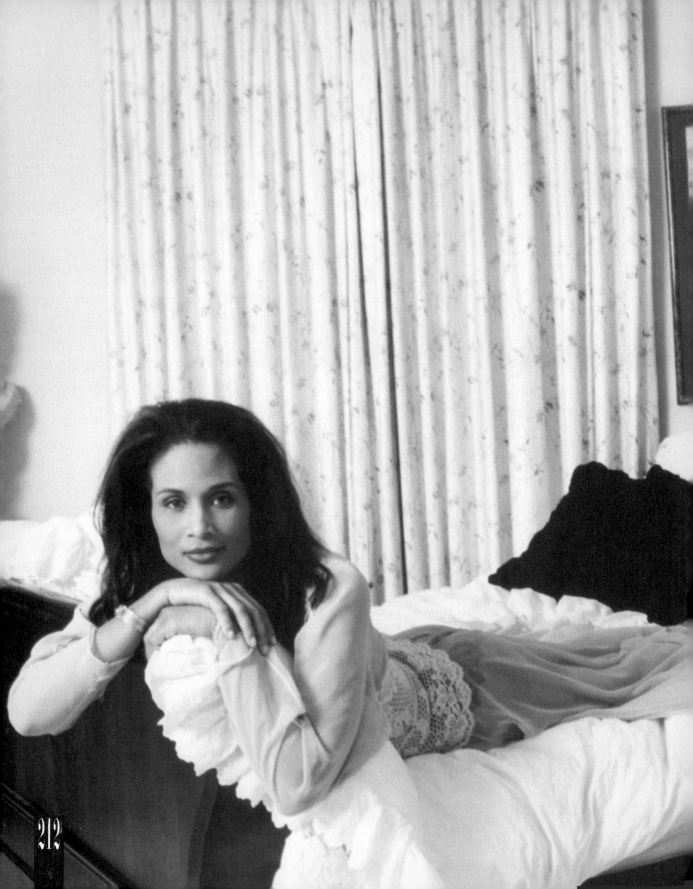

that is so essential to soul-esteem. Or maybe you feel it's just so buried inside of you, so trampled upon since childhood, that you despair of ever reaching it again. To you I say, we've all been there. We've all been put down, disparaged that we're inadequate, that our face is "too this," our hair or our hips "too that."

But the further you get away from soul-esteem, the more strained your relationship becomes with whatever your higher power is, the further away you'll drift from where you want to go.

There will come a point when you will be sick and tired of being sick and tired. From a beauty standpoint, which of course is our focus here, this means being sick and tired of losing and gaining weight, of being bombarded by new, "hot" health and beauty ideas that work for the short term—and then leave you in the very same place you started. Once you've reached that point—and most of us in the 90's are fast approaching it—you'll be ready to move on.

It's at this point that I'm asking you to dig deep down within yourself and pull from that source (and combine it with the tools and techniques that the modern-day beauty industry has to offer). Try it. Reach. You'll feel your soul-esteem stir, then soar. Your beauty, inner and outer—your power—will blossom *as it was meant to be*.

SOLUTIONS: A PLAN FOR SOUL-ESTEEM REJUVENATION

The effect of stress—on work, on our looks and on our health—is hardly a debatable issue anymore. We know that the weight of the pressures we feel is real: too much to do, not enough time, the feeling of having to be in two places (sometimes three places!) at once.

But doing too much can create tension, irritability, and fatigue; it can lead to feelings of failure and depression. Plus, an impossibly tight schedule means that flexibility and spontaneity (and the grace and ease that they bring to your life) are lost.

Private moments alone...that's when you feel your soul-esteem stir...

TIP

Vitamins—what to take, what they do, where they are

Vitamin	Benefits	Natural Sources
Vitamin A	Essential for healthy eyes and skin	Carrots, nuts
Vitamin B-1	Essential for healthy nervous system	Whole grains
Vitamin B-2	Maintains healthy cells and good energy metabolism	Milk, eggs
Vitamin B-3	Maintains normal functioning of body	Chicken, peanuts
Vitamin B-5	Helps energy metabolism, brain function	Whole grains, chicken, fish
Vitamin B-6	Helps body process proteins, fat, and sugar	Wheat germ, fish
Vitamin B-12	Helps maintain healthy blood	Liver, kidneys
Vitamin C	Helps body resist infection, maintains health	Citrus fruits, leafy green vegetables
Vitamin D	Helps body absorb calcium to maintain helthy bones and heart	Sunlight, milk with vitamin D added
Vitamin E	Strengthens immune system, helps body resist disease	Wheat germ, whole grains, vegetable oils

Mineral

Mineral	Benefits	Natural Sources
Calcium	Essential for healthy bones, teeth, and muscles	Dairy products
Chlorine	Helps maintain normal body functioning	Salt, non-bottled water that has been chlorinated
Chromium	Helps sugar metabolism, energizes	Shellfish, whole-wheat bread
Copper	Helps form blood cells, assists vitamin C	Non-bottled water that comes through copper pipes (almost all)
Iodine	Helps maintain normal thyroid function (regulates energy)	Seafood, salt with iodine added
Iron	Helps form blood cells, aids growth	Meat, leafy green vegetables
Magnesium	Helps body utilize all major nutrients	Citrus fruits, apples
Manganese	Helps glands, increases brain function	Bran, leafy green vegetables
Phosphorus	Works with calcium for healthy bones and teeth	Chicken, fish
Potassium	Important for nerve conduction, helps maintain bones and teeth	Bananas, citrus fruits, leafy green vegetables
Selenium	Helps keep tissues elastic, maintains healthy heart	Wheat germ
Zinc	Essential for cell growth, helps protein metabolism	Eggs, whole-wheat bread

Dealing with Stress and Burnout. What to do: Take the time to catch your breath, to slow down. While life is filled with responsibilities (no one is saying you should shirk them), in order to shoulder them effectively, you must make time for recuperation (mental as well as physical), for relaxation, renewal, and repair.

Keep in mind that this is your time to be good to yourself—that you're worth that time, and that it's a journey that's going to be enriching, rewarding, and fun.

HOW TO BEGIN:
STEP 1: BE GOOD TO YOURSELF—IT SHOWS

Think for a moment about what makes you feel good about yourself. What are some of the simple things you can do for yourself to direct your thinking toward the positive? Certainly this can be different things for different people—and certainly women of different ages may find well-being in different ways—working in the garden or roller-skating in the park! Some of us may achieve that sense of personal satisfaction by preparing an incredible meal for our families. Other people (my mother, for one) may experience it by reading, by going to the theater to enjoy a great play, or by traveling to new places. Anansa can sit for hours, dreamily cutting out magazine articles and pictures that intrigue her.

In short, while what's right for a teen of sixteen may hardly appeal to a grandmother of sixty, here are some starting points:

When was the last time you enjoyed a good book? Or tried your hand at writing poetry? Perhaps it's finding the time to plant a garden, to paint, to take a class in modern jazz or ballet, to attend a concert, to try the exhilaration of hiking—wherever your passion lies. I enjoy running on the beach at dawn; I consider it time well spent on myself, for myself, and by myself, and it leaves me calm, yet energized—and better able to cope with whatever each day has to bring. I'm important enough to merit that

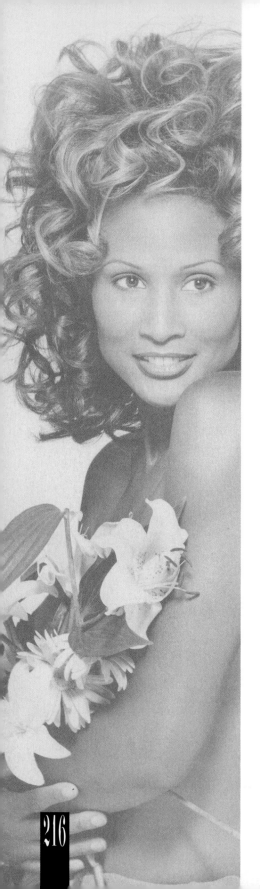

consideration and attention—and you are, too.

Try luxuriating in a scented bath for twenty minutes or so (yes, I know you've heard this before, but there's a reason for that: a soothing soak really can be renewing, for both body and mind). Keeping a diary or journal can help you learn to express your innermost feelings (and writing down problems can often make them more manageable). Or how about putting aside time for the soul-reviving quiet of a half hour of meditation or yoga. Or treating yourself to a stress-relieving, tension-relieving Shiatsu massage.

I believe in surrounding yourself with things of beauty that give you and your loved ones pleasure. This can be as simple as a pot of inexpensive fresh flowers on a bedside table, a fragrant scent perfuming a room, lilting music or caressing textures (a silky robe, pretty pillows). By finding and focusing on the beauty around you, by engaging in positive activities that make you feel good, chances are you'll look better, *too*. The fact is that when you feel good inside, it really does show, in your eyes, your skin, especially in the way you move. And once you begin to view yourself positively—to see the results of treating yourself well, as a human being of worth and value—once you begin to see yourself as a beautiful and vibrant woman, you will begin to tap into that inner beauty source with which every woman is born.

Nothing gives me more pleasure than the beauty of fresh flowers.

TIP

Vitamins

There's nothing exotic about vitamins. Most people take something—whether it's vitamin C to ward off colds in the winter or vitamin E for the skin. The whole idea is to give your body the nutrients you know it needs, but that you miss when you're not able to eat enough to fulfill your daily requirements.

◆

Taking in the calming scent of the sea, the clean smell of sand...we find there's a soul-nurturing quality in this sort of natural aromatherapy.

Once you achieve a sense of center, your inner core begins to respond by radiating beauty to your body, your eyes, your face, your spirit, your soul. Once you start to take control of your life, to feel at ease with who you are and where you are going, that's the sense of beauty—individual, unique, and your own—that you'll project to the world around you. And because there's something inherently appealing, inherently attractive about a person who is comfortable with who she is, you'll become a focal point to which others gravitate.

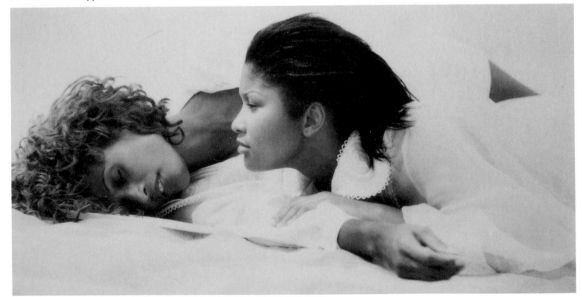

AROMATHERAPY

Flowers on the bedside table, a fragrant perfume scenting the room—this is a start to experiencing the beauty and delight that aromatherapy can bring into your life. I must confess that I've always been interested in the power of fragrance. But more than just pretty, romantic notions of bath oils and scented body lotions, scent can be a trigger—a soothing, calming, healing balm, and a way to release beauty into your life.

Many experts have written that our cultural heritage affects our general attitude toward fragrance—and our personal choice of scents. Some say that darker skin tends to absorb scent and diffuse it less (which may indicate a preference for longer-lasting or stronger scents, often with a musk base). Others tell me that spicy, sultry, Oriental scents are particularly effective on darker-skinned Latin women and African-American women.

My opinion: That the fragrance you choose is truly a matter of individual preference, a personal expression of your own femininity and style—and that it has nothing whatsoever to do with race. I believe that fragrance is a sensual thing, a seductive thing. Unlike some women who have their own "signature" fragrance, I like to try them all (and I especially love to see them beautifully displayed in their sparkling bottles on my dressing table).

Because I am fairly sensitive to fragrances, I tend to change them according to my mood, the time of day, the weather, the season. Sometimes I enjoy a slightly green scent; at other times, I lean toward the heavier florals that are so intensely feminine. Some women like to wear their boyfriend's or husband's fragrances—men's fragrances can be light and citrusy (and of course their scent is entirely different on a woman).

When I go out, I don't consider myself fully dressed until I've applied some fragrance—on my neck, splashed on my chest, on my wrists. Because I try so many different fragrances, I don't really have any favorites. At times I've liked Chanel No. 5 (and I still go back to it), or Joy, Bal de Versailles, Au Savage, Escape, Opium, and

Obsession. But fragrance is so personal. My sister, for example, loves Agnes B., while I associate my mother with White Linen.

Rose fragrances make me feel especially romantic; this is one scent I adore putting in my bath water. I also love scented body lotions, and I frequently mix and layer scents—one lighter, one heavier—to come up with my own combinations.

But understanding the power of scent is more than just this kind of playful experimentation. It's also one more way to bring yourself closer to your dreams. Scent can change your way of thinking. It can alter your perspective, change your direction. It's almost like changing your sleeping position in bed. For example, if you're used to sleeping with your head pointing north, when things aren't going so well try sleeping headed south for a change. You'll find it gives you a different take on things; it opens your mind, so you don't get locked into one position, so to speak.

Well, scent and fragrance are very much like that. It's interesting how scent can trigger memories—how you come to associate different scents with certain events, or people or times in your life. And how one whiff can bring it all rushing back.

Of course, one's reactions to scent are extraordinarily personal (everyone knows how different perfumes and colognes react differently on different people). The scent you love on your mother, sister, or best friend may be totally different on you, as it reacts with your personal body chemistry.

So how can you use scent and aromatherapy to widen your horizons? Why not start in the most simple way by acquiring an appreciation for the unique beauty of many different scents, rather than just one? Open yourself to the sensual pleasure and enjoyment of fragrance in all its forms—and in unexpected places in your life, whether it's in a scented body lotion or a half-hidden candle on a table in your hallway that greets you with subtle fragrance every time you enter your home. Or touch the light bulbs in your room with your favorite scent, so that when you switch on the light, the scent gently permeates the room.

There are other ways to experience the beauty that scent can bring into your life, from delicate sachet pouches of potpourri tucked into your lingerie drawers (release their fragrance with a drop of aromatic oil from time to time) to lemony blocks of cedar wood in your wardrobe, to quilted hangers scented with orange spice in your coat closet, or lavender sprigs and dried vanilla beans tucked among the linens.

One final idea: Put a scented candle by your bedside so that its lingering perfume is the last thing you inhale as you go to sleep. Once you experience the calming, soothing effect it has on your emotions, I think you'll agree that aromatherapy, even in this simplest, most basic way, is an underrated and very powerful thing. And while in and of itself it's a small change, to be sure, it can make a very specific difference in your life by reminding you, with every breeze, every whiff, that you are taking positive care of yourself.

MEDITATION AND AFFIRMATION

Because true beauty calls for you to dig deeper into yourself than you have before—far beyond the superficiality of hair spray and mascara or exercise routines—I also recommend trying meditation as a way to get in touch with your inner core, as a way to center yourself and reach a balance in your life.

In a sense, the kind of meditation I advocate is prayer—not of a religious sort, but rather more spiritual. If that idea makes you feel uncomfortable, think of it as affirmation, a creative visualization of what you want your life to hold, what your goals are, and how to achieve them.

How to: This is how I start and end my days, every morning, early in the morning and every evening before I go to sleep. I want to emphasize that it's not a formalized thing—there are no set prayers or chanting, for example. It's just a special five to ten minutes that I give myself as a gift, a time when I feel consciously in contact with a higher power.

TIP

Herbs for beauty & health

Lychium: Strengthens blood, gives energy, brightens eyes.

◆

Pearl: Clarifies skin, gives skin a deep, luminous shine, clears eyes.

◆

Deer Antler Tips: Cell rejuvenator; restores youthful look to skin.

◆

Ho Shou Wu: Longevity herb. Returns youth, cleanses blood. Increases sperm production in men, fertility in women. Nurtures hair and teeth.

◆

Ginseng (eight different types): Helps body adjust to stress; adapts body's energy to what it needs.

Reishi Mushroom: Heart and blood strengthener. Cleanses system; anti-allergen. Enhances wisdom.

◆

Dragon-Bone: Anti-stress, anti-tension. Stabilizes emotions.

◆

Schizandra: Stabilizes emotions. Clears skin, cleanses system.

◆

Tang Kwei: For women, helps regulate menstrual cycle, improves circulation. For men, aids muscle building.

◆

I achieve this peace through a calming, breathing ritual that most assuredly is not some touchy-feely hocus-pocus. For example, mental exercises similar to this have long been used to relieve stress or to ease chronic pain. Simply lie still, breathing deeply, consciously relaxing each part of your body—your forehead, your neck, your arms and shoulders, your hands and each individual finger, all the way down to your toes. As you focus on doing this (and on breathing deeply), try to clear your mind of all clutter, throwing out your stray thoughts, resting your mind.

If you haven't done this before, I think you'll find that to lie still and focus on breathing is not as simple as it seems. If you're like most people, in fact, your mind will be so cluttered that thoughts, worries, and daily concerns just keep rushing in.

It's important to persist, though, to keep trying, day after day. The effects can only be positive, the effort only worthwhile. Consider this kind of mind control like a muscle. The more you practice this exercise, the easier it's going to become. One day it will work perfectly, and it's going to allow you to achieve an inner stillness that lets you tap into your core. Achieving this allows that essential link between your inner beauty and your outer physical self. Far more than the simple, healthy good sense of de-stressing or relaxing, it's a way to drive your beauty routine to levels that you have never achieved before.

CHINESE HERBALISM

If you've read my previous book on beauty, you'll know that I've long been interested in herbs—I've used them in facial masks, taken them in capsule form, and explored ancient herbal rituals as well as modern ideas of blending herbs to relieve stress, to rejuvenate, and to counteract burnout and anxiety. There are herbs you can take to eliminate a craving for sweets or to cure a sugar addiction. Chamomile is good for headaches; lavender is an excellent mouthwash; comfrey is helpful to asthma sufferers.

The health and beauty benefits of Chinese herbalism has become a particular passion

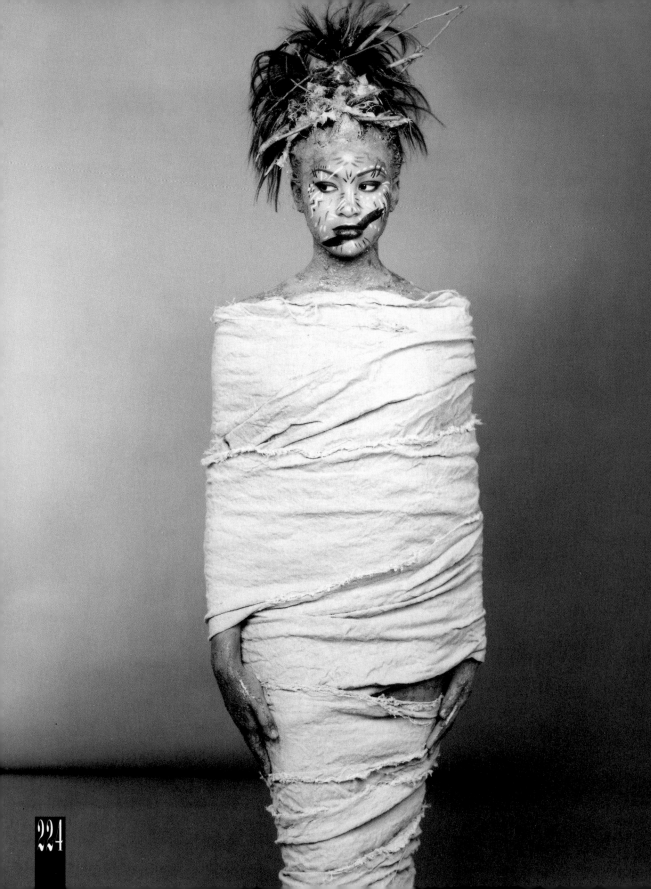

of mine. I became fascinated with Chinese herbs (which one takes in tablet form) shortly after I moved to Los Angeles, and I find that they help my body to function at its optimum, naturally increasing my energy, vitality, and even my creativity, strange as that last may sound to those of you who are unfamiliar with their use.

Although I don't advocate herbs being used medicinally, they have been used for thousands of years to *maintain* health. I found that they helped me overcome a particularly difficult transition in my life: Moving from New York to California involved not only uprooting myself and my daughter, but also changing the focus of my life and career. At that time, I had reached a point where I was so exhausted, both emotionally and physically, by the change that I was ready to try something new.

Chinese herbalism is a way of maintaining good health and well-being through the use of special herbs, taken in pills, teas, and elixirs, and combined with a whole way of life—meditation, yoga, eating well, etc. While Western herbalism uses herbs to cure specific illnesses (a certain tea for a headache, a certain root for a sore throat), Chinese herbalism strives to maintain health by keeping your system in balance, thereby preventing illness before it strikes. Therefore it doesn't emphasize "treating" as much as it does "strengthening." To me, it's all part of living well.

As with everything else associated with the 1960's—from natural products to environmental consciousness—herbalism is all the rage these days. I must stress that I don't regard this as a fad or trend. It has been a way of life for many people for thousands of years.

The secret of Chinese herbalism (and the secret of life) is balance—something I had lost touch with at the time I was introduced to these principles. By keeping all the aspects of your body and life in balance, you'll be better able to maintain good health, productivity, and serenity—all elements that lead to beauty—for all the years of your life.

Every person has three aspects to her being that ideally should be kept in balance.

Be open to new—and old—
ideas...there's lots to be
learned from old-time
remedies. Explore everything—
within reason, that is!

235

They are: "ching," our essence, the body's generator or energy source, if you will; "chi," our day-to-day energy that allows us to move, communicate, and think; and "shen," our spirit, which takes the form of compassion, generosity, and love for ourselves and others. When these three elements are in harmony, health and well-being are achieved.

Many things in our lives can cause us to be out of balance, and you may notice these in yourself. Excessive smoking or drinking, overeating, depression, and stress—all are indications that our lives may be out of balance. Eating disorders, like bulimia, from which I suffered, are a clear indication that something is wrong. Such conditions will most likely lead to physical sickness if left alone. The philosophy behind Chinese herbalism holds that by strengthening our natural resources, we will become less vulnerable to these potentially harmful lifestyles. It involves more than just herbs, too—fresh air, exercise, a good diet, and meditation can all be parts of getting your life in balance.

The herbs themselves can be pure or in mixtures. Each addresses one of the three human aspects. Some herb mixtures help restore the ching, others the chi, others the shen, all in dosages determined by your herbalist. Each person will need a different set of herbs according to what is lacking or out of balance in her life. Because it is so individual, herbalists meet and talk with you before determining your needs. If you suffer from headaches, perhaps they are caused by an imbalance in your shen because you recently lost your job or a good friend. By replenishing your shen with specific herbs rather than giving you an herb that dulls headache pain, you will improve your health and other parts of your life. Or perhaps your insomnia is caused by a depletion of your chi because you've been putting in too much overtime. While there are herbs that will help you sleep, herbs that help restore your chi will also replenish your energy so that you will work more productively and achieve a better balance between work and relaxation time.

When I first met with my herbalist, she could tell that my energy was low because of the move and upheaval I had just gone through. At first, I started taking a regular dose of a specially prepared mixture of herbs, including ginseng. I took three pills every morning and a cup of tea before bed. Almost immediately, I found my energy restored. Over the next few months, my herbalist adjusted the original combination of herbs, adding some, eliminating others, depending not only on my body's needs, but on my mental and emotional needs as well, as my life became more balanced.

These days, whenever I feel particularly run down, I have a special "elixir shake" that is full of ginseng and gives me an incredible boost. But I don't believe in going overboard, and neither should you. I blend herbalism with other things in my life—yoga, meditation, jogging, healthy eating—to keep me totally fit, healthy, and centered.

If you aren't familiar with the benefits of herbalism, why not try it out first in a simple way—a calming herb tea before bed or a pick-me-up ginseng tea before work to make you more awake, more focused. What I find particularly appealing about herbs and their properties is that you feel the effects and reap the benefits immediately. Intrigued? I hope so. Because I truly believe that this is the way for us to learn to heal ourselves, using the best of these time-honored techniques that have been passed down to us from folkloric sources, combined with the knowledge and know-how we have from modern medical and psychological treatments.

♦

SIMPLE TIPS ON HOW TO INCORPORATE THE IDEAS IN THIS CHAPTER INTO YOUR LIFE

Some people associate yoga, meditation, herbalism, and aromatherapy with strange, New Age thinking or bare-footed gurus sitting on top of a mountain, but they are really simple things that we can incorporate into our daily lives to make us calmer, happier, more centered, or more relaxed. Yoga doesn't have to scare you as too spiritual— why not add the stretches to your warm-up or cool-down exercise routine, simply because they feel good. As for meditation, just taking a few minutes for yourself at the end of the day can be a form of meditation. We seldom find any time for ourselves to relax and decompress—and that's all that meditation is. As for aromatherapy, you know how you feel sexy when you put on your favorite fragrance before you go out on a date, or how you feel cozy when you smell something baking? That's armomatherapy right there—the relationship between fragrance and psychology, how different scents affect our moods. Easiest to do (and a body beautifier besides): a few drops of fragrant oil in your bath water (when the water is warm and rushing, the heat and movement help release the scent).

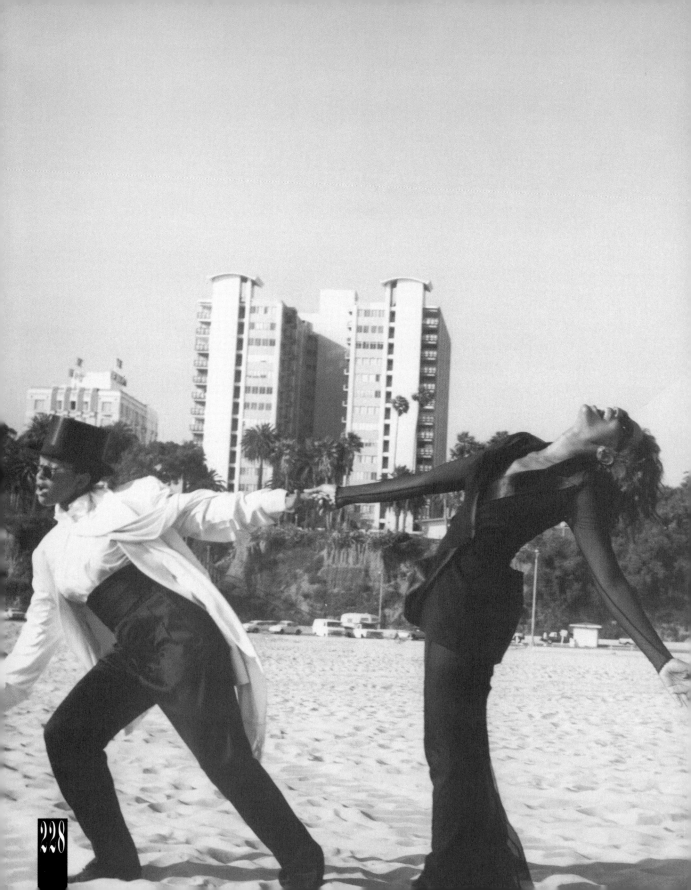

CLOSING

What can I say as this book draws to a close? How can I sum this up? I do believe that being on this planet is an opportunity we're given—a chance to work and improve to become the best we possibly can be. I also believe that inherent in the very idea of true beauty is the idea of a work in progress. We are all continually working, learning, and improving. Beauty, like everything else, is an evolutionary road, and it's one on which we all will eventually find our own way.

If you began this book feeling a bit unhappy or dissatisfied with the way you look, and have come away with some nutritional ideas, some makeup tips, some food for thought, or, even better, a concrete plan to help yourself feel better about your appearance, then I've accomplished some of my initial goals. I truly believe that beauty is an important element in our lives and that it's something to which we're all entitled. Plus, I've found that unhappiness with the way you look—with your face, your body, your hair, superficial as it may sound—can prevent you from reaching your potential in other crucial areas of your life. But I truly believe that learning to integrate practical beauty techniques, nutritious, healthful eating, exercise, positive relationships, and a sense of spiritual balance into your life, will help you achieve a sense of control over and harmony with your own future.

I hope I've managed to provoke some thought: at the most, a new resolve, a new way of looking and perceiving the world around you; at the very least, a new way to put on your mascara. And please let me know if *True Beauty* works for you. I love to hear from women, to learn about their own (sometimes bumpy) path to beauty, because it's a goal we all share—and one we can achieve, besides.

Finally, if I can leave you with one thought, I'd like it to be a thought of love. Once we begin to look at ourselves with loving eyes, we're on our way.

ACKNOWLEDGMENTS

In the course of putting together this book, I've talked with so many different people—doctors and skin-care specialists, top hair and makeup stylists, whose ideas I respect and work I know, trainers, fitness masters, nutritionists and others, melding their advice with what I've learned during my modeling years. I specifically want to acknowledge those people who have so generously contributed their ideas, insights and time to make this book as thorough—and as beautiful—as it can be.

Among those who have been most generous with their time, ideas, and expertise are makeup artists Sam Fine, Fran Cooper, and Joey Mills; Peter Goldman, M.D., associate professor of dermatology; Larry Rosenthal, DDS; plastic surgeon Nicolas Tabbal, M.D., attending surgeon, Manhattan Eye, Ear & Throat Hospital, New York; John Atchison, owner John Atchison Salon, NY; Arlene McCormick, colorist, John Atchison Salon, and especially Heidi Taylor, H. Taylor Concepts & Co., hair stylist and makeup artist, consultant for Lanza and Sebastian products for all her sound information and on-the-spot help. Also, hair stylist Brittannica Stewart; Edward Tricomi, of Edward Tricomi salon; stylist Toni Greene; Allison Terry for her thoughts on weaving, extensions and hair buying; Olive Benson, owner, Olive's Beauty Salon, Boston; Jennifer Stack, R.D.N., registered dietitian and senior nutritionist at New York University Medical Center; nutritionist Joanne Smith of Healthy Image, LA; Keith Byard, fitness trainer/owner Physique Rio, NY; New York trainer and fitness expert Lynn Letts; Samy Suarez, owner of Samy Suarez Salon Systems in Miami; Salon Ishi in NY; Josephine

Hawley-Allen at Atelier de Beaute Salon; psychotherapist Dana Dovitch, Ph.D.; Jane Cooper, C.S.W, M.S.E.d, exercise physiologist and social worker. New York trainer Binky Brooks, Vanderbilt YMCA; herbalist Susan Haffey at Ron Teaguarden, LA; researchers Nancy Stillpass, Marie Luise Proeller and Suzanne Undy.

I also want to thank everyone at Warner Books who believed in this book, including Larry Kirshbaum, Maureen Egen, Karen Kelly, and Jeanmarie LeMense. Very special appreciation to Vickie Peslak Hyman and her creative design team at Platinum Design, for working so hard (and *succeeding!*) in making this book as beautiful as it can be, and to Allison Kyle Leopold for helping me express not only the words that were in my head but the love that is in my heart.

Special thanks, too, to Jimmy Hester, and to photographer Patrick Demarchelier and all the glorious women of color who appear in this book; also to diet guru Nikki Haskell and to some very special friends—Matilda Cruz, my second mother; Sandy Hart and Yvonne (Dada) Bratton, my best friends forever; and my dear, dear friend and fellow model Janice Dickinson.

Finally, to my own family—whom I am grateful to and thankful for every day of my life: to the memory of my father for his amazing cheekbones, his color and his guidance; for my mother Gloria Johnson, for her grace and beauty; my younger brother Darren, a New York City therapist who encourages and loves me...and makes me love myself; my baby sister Joanne for her unconditional love and admiration; my big brother Leon, who got me hooked on exercise by insisting that if Cher can have a good body so could I. All my love always to my daughter Anansa, my best fashion and beauty consultant and confidante; and to my big sister Sheila Wright, a teacher and therapist, who told me way back in 1988 to go and write this book—my thanks.

—Beverly Ann Johnson

CREDITS:

Grateful acknowledgment is made to the following for permission to use photographs:

Mark Abrahams: Pages 1, 5, 35, 46

Jaramy Aref: Pages 23, 50

Marc Baptiste: Pages 6, 20, 155, Chapter 6 Opener, 189, 198-9, 202

Charles William Bush: Pages 22, 130

Gregory Cannon: Pages 2, 4, 5, Chapter 2 Opener, 33, 37, 41, 47, 101, 106, 137-9, 201, 211, 230-1

Indira Cesarine: Pages 64-65, 162, 180, Chapter 7 Opener

Michel Comte: Pages 179, 218, 228

Patrick Demarchelier: Cover Title Page, 52, 60, 142-3, 192-3, 216-7, 231

Janice Dickenson: Pages 8, 10, 19, 72, 75-7, 108, 112, 125, 142-7, 158, 174, 184, 190, 194

Bob Elias: Pages 70, 88, Chapter 4 Opener, 109, 120, Part II Opener

Gerard Gentil: Pages 24, 104

Michel Haddi/ *Visages*: Pages 42, 115

Brad Hahn: Pages 38, 56-7, 140-1

Adrian Houston: Pages 14, Chapter 5 Opener, 212

Catalina Leisenring/ *Tatoo Fotography Management*: Pages 9, 146-7

Roxanne Lowit: Pages 93, 128, 230-1

Patrick McMullin: Page 230

Amyn Nasser/ *Tatoo Fotography Management:* Pages 79-82

Andy Pearlman: Pages 49, 116, 156, 171, 188, 195

Len Prince: Chapter 3 Opener, 224

Bonnie Schiffman: Pages 13, 164

Sandy Simpson: Part I Opener, Chapter 1 Opener, 30, 44-5, 63, 117, 148

Viviane Ventura: Pages 96, 123, 131, 136, 230

Grateful acknowledgment is also made to the following for makeup, hair, styling, and assisting:

Edgar Ceav

Angelo DiBiase

Charles Dujic/Celestine

Lauren Ehrenfeld/Celestine

Kris Evans

Andreo Fagndes

Mel Grayson

Teri Groves

Justin Henry

Rachel London

Didi Malique

Anne Marso

Joseph Oppedisano